Paleo Grilling offers amazing tools that help to bring families back to the dinner [table] with food that nourishes not only the body but relationships as well. There's not [nothing?] creations: the smells that waft in through open windows in late summer, the soun[d] and people laughing and enjoying each other's company. *Paleo Grilling* is more than just another cook[book]. a way to encourage your loved ones to gather together, thanks to the joy of real food. And your kids just might forget for at least one evening that processed food even exists.

   —**Sarah Fragoso, everydaypaleo.com and eplifefit.com**

Paleo Grilling begins by weaving a beautifully written historical perspective of how the innovation of meat to fire sent us on a course toward what we call human, and the cost and consequences of convenience. The story develops full circle to arrive at the Paleo, slow food, and locavore movements of today—seeking something more deep and meaningful in how we nourish ourselves.

Tony Federico and Chef James Phelan set out to help us do just that: teaching us all about sourcing our food, what it means to cook nose-to-tail, how to grill to perfection, all while sharing their masterfully crafted, delicious looking recipes. Ultimately however, *Paleo Grilling* is about seeking maximum nutrition with minimal impact by connecting with our past, celebrating our present, and creating hope for our future.

   —**Diane Sanfilippo,** *New York Times* **best-selling author of** *Practical Paleo*

With beautiful photos, helpful how-to's, and mouthwatering recipes, *Paleo Grilling* will inspire you to eat healthy whether you follow a Paleo diet or not.

   —**Elana Amsterdam,** *New York Times* **best-selling author of** *Paleo Cooking from Elana's Pantry*

For all negative press that meat has received in recent years, the fact is that it's a naturally healthy part of the human diet. Some would even say that it's the perfect food, providing all the fat, protein, and micronutrients the human body could ever need when you eat the whole animal. That's what Paleo and meat enthusiasts Tony Federico and James Phelan explore thoroughly in *Paleo Grilling*, providing plenty of recipes that are perfect for a low-carb, high-fat, ketogenic, and Paleo diets.

   —**Jimmy Moore, author of** *Cholesterol Clarity* **and** *Keto Clarity*, **LivinLaVidaLowCarb.com**

I'm a grill-in-every-season kind of girl and I seem to have met my distant grilling cousins in authors Tony Federico and James Phelan. Their respect for the beauty of humanely raised meat and fire shows on every page. With recipes for luscious sauces and meaty meals, they've got your grilling staples covered. But there are also unexpected ways to use the grill in dishes like blackened caesar salad and smoky mushroom soup so you can fire up your grill all year long.

   —**Melissa Joulwan, author of** *Well Fed 2: More Paleo Recipes for People Who Love to Eat* **and**
     TheClothesMakeTheGirl.com

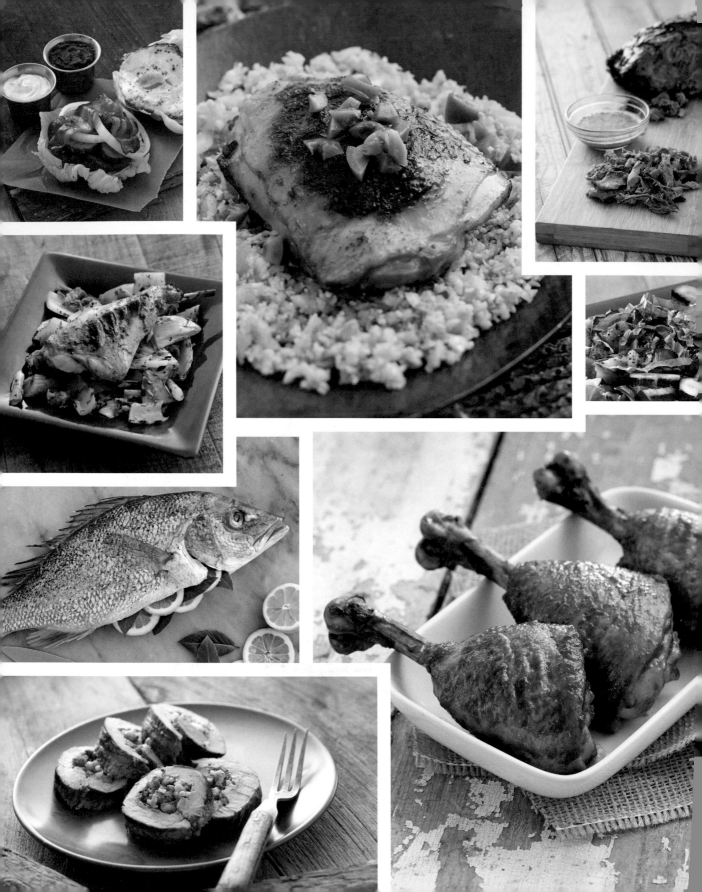

PALEO GRILLING

A MODERN CAVEMAN'S GUIDE TO COOKING WITH FIRE

Tony Federico, A.C.S.M. Health and Fitness Specialist
and Chef James Phelan
Foreword by Amy Kubal, Registered Dietitian

Fair Winds Press
100 Cummings Center, Suite 406L
Beverly, MA 01915

fairwindspress.com • quarryspoon.com

© 2014 Fair Winds Press

First published in the USA in 2014 by
Fair Winds Press, a member of
Quarto Publishing Group USA Inc.
100 Cummings Center
Suite 406-L
Beverly, MA 01915-6101
www.fairwindspress.com
Visit www.QuarrySPOON.com and help us celebrate food and culture
one spoonful at a time!

18 17 16 15 14   1 2 3 4 5

ISBN: 978-1-59233-612-8

Digital edition published in 2014
eISBN: 978-1-62788-027-5

Library of Congress Cataloging-in-Publication Data available

   Federico, Tony.
    Paleo grilling : a modern caveman's guide to cooking with fire / Tony Federico
and James W. Phelan.
      pages cm
   Includes index.
   ISBN 978-1-59233-612-8
   1. Reducing diets--Recipes. 2. High-protein diet. 3. Prehistoric peoples-
-Nutrition. I. Phelan, James W. II. Title.
   RM222.2.F394 2014
   641.5'638--dc23

                                             2014004446

Cover and book design by The Lincoln Avenue Workshop
Photography by Glenn Scott Photography
Styling by Jen Beauchesne

Printed and bound in China

*The information in this book is for educational purposes only. It is not
intended to replace the advice of a physician or medical practitioner. Please
see your health care provider before beginning any new health program.*

To my beautiful wife, Jamie, for her unfailing support, patience, and ability to keep me focused on what's most important. To my brother from another mother, Tim Bryant, who talked me into doing this book in the first place and who encouraged me to "Keep on chopping!" To my mom, for her irrational belief in me. To my dad, for teaching me the value of hard work and perseverance. To my sister, for reminding me that I'm not "the f'n Buddha." To Doug Baggett, for changing my life by giving me a copy of Loren Cordain's *The Paleo Diet.* To all the amazing staff and members at the Deerwood Country Club Fitness Center. And last but not at all least, to my friends in the Paleo community who constantly inspire me with their books, blogs, photography, podcasts, and passion. If I have done something of worth here, "it is by standing on the shoulders of giants."

—Tony Federico

It is my sincere hope that every one of you has a love in your life like the one I have for my wife, Britt. My contributions to this book are dedicated to her.

—James "Jay" Phelan

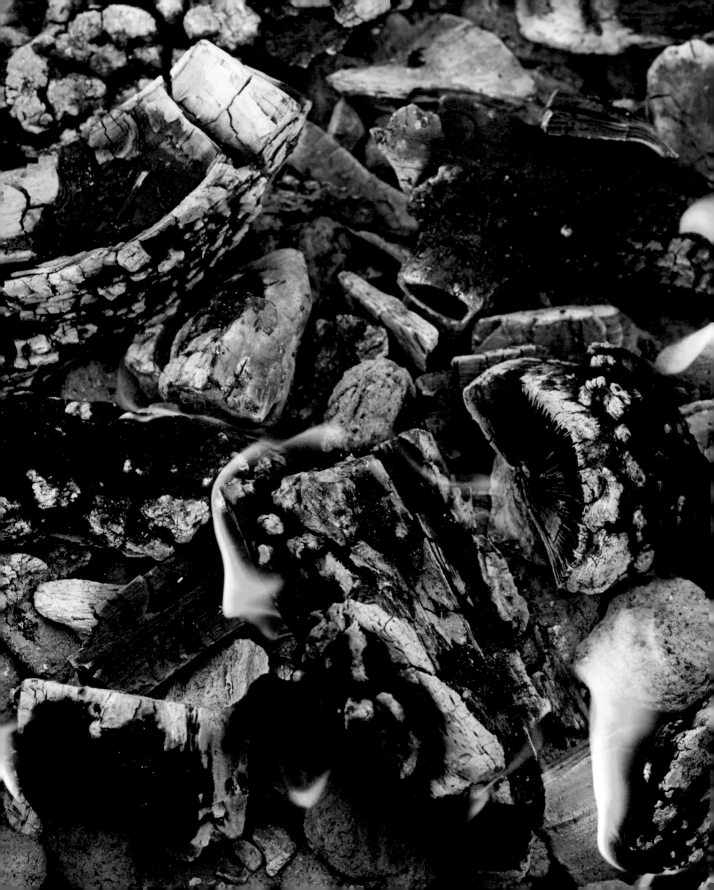

CONTENTS

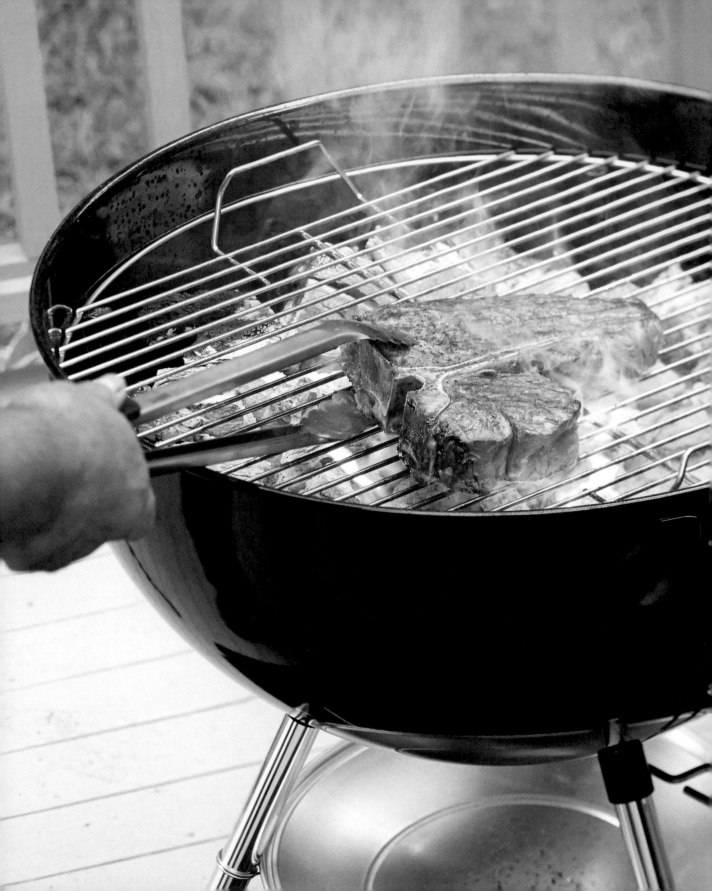

FOREWORD

BY AMY KUBAL, R.D., L.D.

Paleo Grilling encourages us to think, live, and eat like modern cavemen. Eating meat, vegetables, nuts, seeds, and fruit while sitting around the campfire was the caveman's lifestyle. Simple. But in today's hustle and bustle convenience is king, where fast food, buffets, mega-supermarkets, and easy-to-access food are commonplace. If modern humans actually had to hunt and gather our food in order to eat and survive, our diets would naturally look much different—and much simpler.

One thing we recognize about our convenience-oriented food environment is that it's making us sick. Obesity, diabetes, heart disease, autoimmune conditions, and many other diet- and lifestyle-related health problems are on the rise. The effects of eating simpler, real food as a means to combat these health issues is one of the many reasons the Paleo diet has become so popular. The Paleo eating style has the ability to prevent and reverse many disease processes, enhance athletic performance, and increase quality of life. Sticking to the basics of grass-fed or lean meats, vegetables, healthy fats, and moderate amounts of fruits, nuts, and seeds will do far more for our health than anything that comes out of a drive-through window.

Cooking for yourself on a regular basis and living a full Paleo lifestyle will take more thought, attention, and time, but your health is worth it—and eating Paleo tastes pretty damn good, too. There are many great ways to prepare meats and vegetables, and this book provides one that doesn't require turning on the oven or scrubbing a bunch of pans. Grilling is an excellent way to prepare delicious Paleo meals for you and your family even when you're short on time. And who doesn't love a backyard barbecue?

Despite its title, this book is about much more than throwing meat on the fire. This book encourages a Paleo lifestyle that means what you eat is fuel—whether you're doing chores around the house all day or preparing for an epic CrossFit workout. Real, healthy food equals real, healthy energy. The Paleo lifestyle means avoiding processed foods in favor of natural ingredients, and this book shows you how to make your own condiments, spices, sauces, and marinades from scratch with the freshest, best ingredients (so you can skip the store-bought mayo and ketchup). And Paleo is more than just meat—this cookbook includes recipes for Paleo-friendly drinks, salads, soups, starters, and desserts.

So let's not waste any more time. Put your apron on, grab your spatula and tongs, fire up the grill, and get ready to dig into some "meaty" Paleo recipes and meals!

ABOUT AMY KUBAL

Amy Kubal is a registered and licensed dietitian specializing in the Paleo diet and performance nutrition. She is the consulting dietitian for Robb Wolf and the director of Robb's Paleo R.D. Network. Additionally, she is the nutrition guru for the Whole9 and Joe Friel's TrainingBible coaching. Amy has helped many clients optimize body composition and manage and recover from autoimmune and diet-related diseases: cancer, diabetes, heart disease, irritable bowel syndrome, renal failure, lupus, and more. She works with a broad range of performance-focused clients made up of Olympic athletes, Ironman triathletes, professional bikers, marathoners, CrossFit games competitors, mixed martial arts (MMA) fighters, kettle-bell masters, and everyday athletes.

THE HISTORY OF MEAT AND FIRE

"Somewhere close behind air and water is the need for food." **—L. J. MARTIN,** *Cooking Wild & Wonderful*

THE FIRST TASTE

Charred, blackened, and cooked, the morsel was brought to the mouth and chewed, contemplated, and swallowed with relish. There was no sauce or seasoning and no consideration for aesthetics or art. Yet the combination of meat and fire yielded something revolutionary. Cooked meat made man happy.

This first taste of cooked flesh by an ancient relative of modern humans might have come courtesy of an unlucky animal caught in a wildfire and happened upon by an early hominid. Or it may have been prepared intentionally, the result of a primitive chef who, in the attempt to craft a stone tool, learned that certain stones yielded sparks, and that sparks conjured flames, and by flames, tough and unyielding meat could be turned into something different, something desirable. How we embarked upon this transformation, one that carried us from the realm of animal into that of human isn't exactly clear, but there is evidence, both archeological and biological, that give clues as to how it may have occurred.

MAN THE HUNTER

There are ancient bones, some as old as 3.4 million years, that bear the marks of cutting, scraping, and crushing. This wasn't the work of modern humans, who appeared approximately 200,000 years ago. The credit for this first act of culinary butchery would have to be given to *Australopithecus afarensis*. *Australopithecus* became famous with the discovery of "Lucy," a 3.2-million-year-old hominid skeleton found in Ethiopia. Lucy is thought to have walked upright, leaving her hands free to carry food and perhaps to fashion tools, an important trait for a primitive chef.

If you have ever tried to butcher an animal yourself, you know that tearing one apart barehanded is not a realistic task. Tendons and ligaments are designed to be tough and to withstand great forces; they don't concede their hold without a fight. However, at the hands of a skilled butcher, and a sharp knife, a huge carcass can be broken down in minutes. During Lucy's time, metal tools would have been unimaginable, but with flakes of stone serving as knives, *A. afarensis* would have been able to quickly shear flesh and smash open bones, efficiently extracting fatty marrow and protein-rich flesh.

Whether they acquired meat by hunting or by scavenging the remains of other animals' kills, human ancestors were now in direct competition with some seriously nasty predators, including large cats, crocodiles, and even prehistoric eagles. In competing with these animals we would have had to use cunning to avoid becoming dinner ourselves. Even our prey, antelope and the like, were not to be trifled with. The idea that we evolved with hunting, and that this act shaped us as much as we shaped the world, is commonly referred to as the "Man the Hunter" hypothesis. As hunters we would trade large stomachs, useful for eating vegetables, for large brains, useful for managing the complexities of the kill.

MAN THE COOK

If you look at the human family tree, you can see that progress was made in fits and starts. While there was a considerable increase in brain size from the inclusion of meat in our diets at the time of Lucy, this growth remained relatively stagnant for several million more years. It wasn't until the appearance of *Homo habilis* approximately 1.8 million years ago that our brains embarked on their current exponential growth. As compelling as it might be, the "Man the Hunter" hypothesis is hard-pressed to explain this strange lag. If it were true that animal foods and the social demands of hunting were the sole stimulus for our development of big brains, then we would expect to see brain size increasing much sooner.

"It is by fire that man has tamed Nature itself."
—JEAN-ANTHELME BRILLAT-SAVARIN

An apparent answer to this puzzle comes by way of Harvard University professor of biological anthropology, Richard Wrangham. Wrangham hypothesized that the consumption of raw animal flesh can explain some of the advances in brain size seen by our early ancestors, but the real innovation, the one that sent us on a course toward what we call human, came when we introduced meat to fire. But what's so important about cooking, and why would it cause such a drastic change?

Observing a group of chimpanzees, you would notice a few key things. First, their groups tend to cover large areas, necessary so that they can acquire sufficient amounts of ripe fruit that tends to mature on different trees at different times. Second, when they do discover fruit, it is typically fibrous and difficult to chew, making it necessary for chimps to spend a considerable amount of time masticating their food. In fact, as much as 48 percent of a chimp's day is devoted to chewing. Modern humans, by comparison, spend as little as 4.7 percent of their time chewing, and often less if they are in a hurry.

Animal parts, especially the organs, relative to fibrous fruits and vegetation, are considerably easier to chew. Even chimps, who only consume about 2 percent of their diet from animal sources, go right for the guts when they make a kill. Even so, raw meat is still quite toothsome. It is worth remembering that a prehistoric menu wouldn't have featured tender cuts of domesticated cattle; rather, it would have been made up of antelope and other wild game. Yet humans show a distinct trend toward small mouths, small teeth, and weak jaws. We don't have the sharp, shearing jaws of true carnivores like lions and hyenas. This is where fire comes in.

Cooking softens meat by breaking down the tough connective tissues. What was once stringy and tough becomes succulent thanks to a chemical process called denaturation. Heat denatures proteins by causing the molecules to move so violently that their basic structure is changed. Denatured proteins, in addition to being more easily chewed, are more easily digested because enzymes in the stomach have a greater surface area upon which to act. This translates into a twofold benefit, with less energy required for chewing and digesting and thus more energy extracted from the food itself. Of course, early humans didn't think, "Hmm, cooked meat is more digestible and efficient!" Their taste buds, like ours, were simply wired to detect these benefits and to translate them into sensations of deliciousness.

LIKE MOTHS TO A FLAME

Without question, we are simply attracted to cooked meat like a beef roast, richly browned on the outside with the promise of tender strands inside; sweet and salty, crispy bacon; or flaky fish, with a golden skin. The smell lures us in, beckoning to our senses, "Come closer, there are good things here."

The first primitive cooks knew instinctively that cooked food was tasty, and they grew strong bodies and cunning minds in the many thousands of generations eating meat in the wild. At what stage this cooking took the form of art we may never know, but as humankind developed, so did our culinary skills.

Approximately 15,000 years ago in the region of modern-day Iraq, a great upheaval occurred when humans began domesticating plants. Wild cereal grasses were sown and reaped, yielding greater quantities of food than could be had by the traditional way of hunting and gathering. As it so happened, there were also animals that could be cajoled into captivity, bred into docility, and raised for our eating. The first domesticated

"Human beings do not eat nutrients, they eat food." —**MARY CATHERINE BATESON**

animals were a boon to ancient humans. By transforming grass, shrubs, and other inedible vegetable matter into meat, milk, and eggs, domesticated animals became walking larders, refrigerators on legs.

Perhaps it was then, when man began to separate himself further from the other beasts, by creating rather than finding food, by bending nature to his will rather than surrendering to it, that he, or she, emerged as the first professional cook. Surely there were individuals skilled in the preparation of food long before this time. Hunter-gatherer people possessed all the creative and intellectual skills of the early agriculturalists, perhaps even more so due to their more egalitarian societies where each man, woman, and child needed to be a master of survival. But, in the age of agriculture, society, like the human body itself, divided and specialized.

Because enough food for the many could be produced by a few, classes and trades emerged. The shaman was replaced by the priesthood, the lone trader became a horde of merchants, the tribal chief gave way to royalty and nobility, and the family fire became the kitchen. Man continued to expand across the globe, and in this expansion, new plants and animals were brought to the menu, transformed by fire, and set upon the table. Spices traveled between the Far East and Europe, tomatoes and potatoes crossed between the New World and the Old, and wars and conquests created the food traditions celebrated today.

Walking down a typical suburban street, we can see the product of humanity's violent expansions and contractions. Like waves crashing back upon the ocean, we spread out across the globe only to fall back into ourselves. Shish kebab, literally "skewered meat," hails from the Middle East and Mediterranean region. Barbecue, a derivation of the word *barbacoa*, which translates as "sacred fire pit," comes to us from the Taino people of the Caribbean. Strips of meat, seared over coals, coaxed by fanning to white-hot heat, are products of the Japanese hibachi, or "fire bowl."

THE COST OF CONVENIENCE

The history of meat and fire is intricately woven into the history of mankind itself, from the first awkward graspings of an *Australopithecus* to the refined swipe of a chef's blade. We are culinary creatures at our very core. Yet a peculiar thing has been happening as of late, one that has implications rivaling the great upheavals of fire and agriculture: the curse of convenience.

"We may find in the long run that tinned food is a deadlier weapon than the machine gun." **—GEORGE ORWELL**

Throughout the latter part of the twentieth century, corporations have been elbowing between us and our kitchens. Meat that would have been raised in your town, cooked by the hand of a relative, and shared among friends is now slaughtered in a distant land, prepared by machines, and warmed by a microwave. We have given up our connection to food, the animals, the plants, and the people for a few extra minutes of time, time that we are likely spending in front of a TV or with a computer or smartphone. It would seem as though the story of meat and fire has come to a sad end—but all is not lost.

MEAT AND FIRE FOREVER!

Across the globe people are rediscovering the delights of local food. They are getting back into the kitchen, taking an interest in where their food comes from and how it was raised, and they might even be raising it themselves. The Paleo, locavore, and slow-food movements all speak to a similar hunger, one that casts off convenience for something deeper and more meaningful. Meat and fire, our primal recipe for sustenance, will live on, not as a necessity but as a choice.

Remember this: Each time we marry an impeccably sourced slab of meat with a hot open flame, share it among friends and family, and give thanks for the nourishment it provides, we connect with our past, celebrate our present, and create hope for our future.

MEET YOUR MEAT

There are few foods as contentious as meat. News headlines frequently flash warnings that eating meat is dangerous, is toxic, and will kill you quicker than a saber-toothed tiger bite. Others cite the abhorrent conditions of factory farms and the inhumane treatment of livestock. For years we've been told that meat has too much cholesterol and too much saturated fat, is carcinogenic, and contributes to high blood pressure.

Plant-based diets are touted as both healthier and more sustainable. Critics of carnivory argue that meat production uses up too much of our natural resources and cow farts are responsible for global warming. If what the critics say is true, that meat is bad for our health and bad for the planet, why does the Paleo community support meat but not wheat?

IS MEAT EATING HEALTHY?

On an intuitive level, we all crave meat. Even devout vegetarians and vegans have been known to cheat when confronted with a sizzling slice of bacon. Frankly, meat is delicious. There are few foods that inspire such passion, dedication, and affection as meat.

"If it has four legs and it's not a table, eat it." **—CANTONESE SAYING**

We can be certain that our prehistoric ancestors ate meat. We have the marks on ancient animal bones to prove it. Eating other animals provided early humans with a rich source of usable calories that may have allowed us to become the big-brained clever creatures we are today, but the question of whether or not something is "Paleo" should really take a backseat to whether or not a food is healthful, causing a minimal amount of harm for a maximum amount of benefit.

What the Paleo perspective does is help us understand how food has influenced humanity from a historical, ecological, and evolutionary perspective. You don't have to be a scientist to see the changes that are taking place in our society. The average American's diet is vastly different than it was only a generation ago, processed foods and packaged foods have displaced whole fruits, vegetables, and meats, and as a result, we are fatter and sicker than ever before. Health care costs are skyrocketing, hospitals and pharmaceutical companies are booming, and many of us are suffering from chronic diseases. Looking at the way ancient peoples ate gives us the perfect framework for determining what we can do better.

DEFINING MEAT

If you were to take a peek at the plate of an average American, what is called "meat" would likely be a piece of skeletal muscle. This muscle meat typically comes free of bones and skin, trimmed of excess fat, tidily contained in a clear plastic wrapper, and "hunted" from your grocery store's meat aisle. To a prehistoric human, however, hunting for meat was a matter of survival. A successful hunt would have been celebrated, and not even the smallest scrap would have been wasted. Bones could be fashioned into weapons, tools, and jewelry, or smashed open for their rich marrow; skins could be made into clothing; and everything else would have been eaten. We don't even have to travel all the way back to the Paleolithic era to find cultures that embrace whole-animal eating as a way of life.

In contemporary Mexican cuisine you'll find menudo soup made with tripe (beef stomach) and *tacos de lengua* made from braised beef tongue. In the Philippines you might be served *bopis* (sautéed pig lung) as part of a tapas-style meal. The Scottish are fond of haggis, a boiled sheep's stomach stuffed with "pluck" (sheep's heart, liver, and lungs) and the English have black pudding, which isn't a pudding but rather a sausage filled with congealed blood. Even here in America liver and onions was until very recently a dinnertime staple.

The nutrients provided by organ meats, known collectively as "offal," include high concentrations of fat-soluble vitamins, minerals, and cofactors that aren't present in muscle tissue. Eating things such as skin, tendon, and cartilage provides the amino acids glycine and proline, which

Purchase grass-fed and grass-finished beef whenever possible.

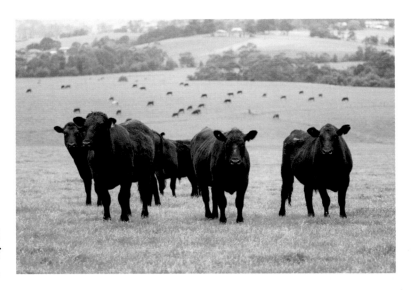

support the body's own ability to generate connective tissue. From a dietary perspective, eating from the whole animal provides a tremendous diversity of nutrients that you will never get if you only eat lean muscle meat. In addition to having a limited definition of meat, most consumers are limited in terms of the types of animals that they eat, sticking to a familiar few species.

According to the American Meat Institute, in 2011 U.S. meat producers generated 26.3 billion pounds of beef, 22.8 billion pounds of pork, 5.8 billion pounds of turkey, and an astonishing 37.7 billion pounds of chicken. In a distant fourth place, with a combined total of 291 million pounds, were veal, lamb, and mutton that went to market. This represents a grand total of five species. To get an idea of how this stacks up to our Paleolithic ancestors, we can look at coprolites, a fancy term for fossilized poop, to see exactly what they were eating.

In a study of coprolites found in Texas caves occupied by between the years of 7000 BCE to about 1000 CE, researchers found the following bones: ringtail cat, coyote (or possibly dog), beaver, kangaroo, rat, porcupine, painted turtle, ground squirrel, pocket gopher, gar fish, sucker fish, marmot, wood rat, deer, elk, jack rabbit, bighorn sheep, horned lizard, raccoon, catfish, frog, spiny lizard, spotted skunk, soft-shell turtle, dove, fox, and insects. There were even more animals on the list, but I think you get the point. Although the exact animals featured on an ancient hunter-gatherer's menu would have varied, if the environment allowed, they would have dined on dozens if not hundreds of species!

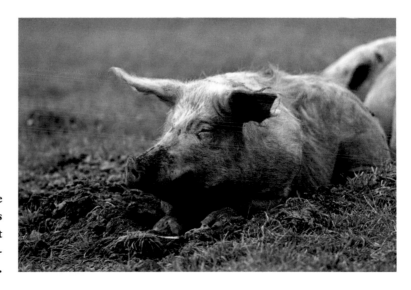

Pastured pork may sometimes be fed grain, but their lifestyle is much healthier and their meat much tastier than their conventionally raised counterparts.

The wild species that prehistoric man hunted, fished, speared, and seared over open flames weren't docile farm animals. These creatures were highly trained athletes, they were on the move, they were hunting and they were hunted, they were predators and prey. Even the ancestral equivalents of cows, chickens, and pigs were a far cry from the fat feedlot-raised steers, big-breasted broiler chickens, and penned-up porkers that make up much of the American meat market. They didn't require constant dosing with antibiotics, and they certainly weren't pumped full of growth hormones, steroids, and antibiotics. It was also pretty unlikely that they would dine on genetically modified corn, soybean meal, and plastic pellets.

The bottom line is that meat eating in the Paleolithic era meant nose-to-tail consumption of a wide variety of wild animals. By comparison, meat eating today often means eating only a few parts from a small number of sick, chemically enhanced animals. When discussing the advantages and disadvantages of eating meat, we should take this fundamental difference into consideration. Yet, studies of meat consumption that seemingly "prove" that meat is unhealthy rarely do this.

THE CHINA STUDY

If you've ever talked to a vegan or seen the movie *Forks Over Knives,* you've probably heard of *The China Study,* a book by Cornell University professor T. Colin Campbell. In *The China Study,* Campbell concludes that the consumption of animal-based foods increases the risk for numerous cancers and chronic diseases. At first glance, it seems like an open and shut case—if you eat meat you'll raise your cholesterol levels and increase your chance of getting cancer—but digging deeper, the story becomes much less convincing.

Nutrition researcher Chris Masterjohn dissected the data presented in *The China Study* and found that "sugar, soluble carbohydrates, and fiber all have correlations with cancer mortality about seven times the magnitude of that with animal protein, and total fat and fat as a percentage of calories were both negatively correlated with cancer mortality." In other words, the real conclusion that Campbell should have presented is to avoid eating too much refined sugars and carbohydrates. Masterjohn also identifies how Campbell demonstrates a clear bias against animal foods, implicating milk proteins in the development of autoimmune diseases such as diabetes, but ignoring the possible contribution of the problematic proteins found in wheat.

Separate studies that seem to indict meat eating as a cause of cancer typically grab headlines, but these hastily produced news stories tend to leave out some important facts. The highest risk of cancer seems to be related to eating "processed" meats and fresh meat consumption poses a much lower risk. None of these studies has focused on an ancestral diet where many different animals are consumed in nose-to-tail fashion along with whole plant foods. The meat eaters in these studies are also consuming large amounts of refined grains, sugars, and other foods that are known to directly contribute to metabolic disease and could likely make meat eating more risky than it would be in the ancestral model.

Although long-term studies of modern people following the Paleo approach have not been conducted, there is ample evidence that suggests that eating like our ancestors did will not promote diseases like cancer and diabetes. This evidence comes from the study of modern hunter-gatherer groups that retained their cultural traditions well into the twentieth century. Their diets of wild game and uncultivated vegetables were likely very similar to that of our prehistoric ancestors, and it is precisely this sort of diet that is advocated by the Paleo approach. Most hunter-gatherer societies derived more than 50 percent of their daily calories from animal products, with higher daily protein intakes and higher cholesterol intakes than that of modern Americans.

Despite what people like T. Colin Campbell claim, the meat-heavy diets of hunter-gatherers did not lead to epidemics of cardiovascular disease, cancer, diabetes, and other related conditions. In fact, even in groups that subsisted almost entirely on animal products, like the Inuit, these diseases were almost nonexistent. It was only after sugar and white flour displaced traditional foods that indigenous peoples began to suffer from Western diseases.

There are some who suggest that hunter-gatherers have special genetic traits that protect them from the "damaging" effects of meat consumption, and this may be part of the story, but a much simpler explanation is that fresh, whole meat products from wild animals are perfectly healthy and, along with nutrient-dense plants, represent the perfect diet for humans. Unfortunately, most of us neither have the skill nor the time to hunt and gather all of our food. The good news is that you can still derive most of the benefits of eating wild without learning how to throw a spear—although you probably should learn how to throw a spear because that would be pretty cool.

SMALL, LOCAL FARMS

Although a diet of wild animals and uncultivated plants represents the ideal, the next best thing is to find sources of responsibly raised domesticated animals. Looking at the packaging in your local supermarket, you will see pictures that suggest that all the cows, chickens, and pigs are living together on cute farms with red barns, but the truth, as you know, is much different. The food industry uses deceptive marketing to hide the fact that their animals live in factories rather than fields, and even labels such as "organic" and "free range" have been corrupted. The solution, then, is to meet your meat. Literally.

A simple Internet search will likely reveal that right outside of your city or town there are small producers who are in dire need of customers.

"Shake the hand that feeds you." **—MICHAEL POLLAN**

(If you live in an area where there aren't any options for responsibly raised local meat, there are excellent mail-order vendors that ship good meat across the country. For a list of some of these vendors, check out the Resources section on page 171.) The little family farms that currently make up only a fraction of the modern meat industry lack the marketing and infrastructure of multinational conglomerates such as ConAgra and Archer Daniels Midland, but what they lack in market share they make up for in passion and care for what they do. Granted, there are local farms that feed their animals GMO (genetically modified organisms) grains, use antibiotics, or treat their animals poorly, but they have less to gain and more to lose from those practices.

Most small farmers live right on their land, so it is in their own best interests to use practices that keep the land healthy. They raise smaller numbers of animals, so they are motivated to take good care of each and every one. They can't afford to simply write off "downer" cows as a cost of doing business, like a concentrated animal feeding operation (CAFO) can. Small farmers also frequently interact with their customers, either directly, at farmers' markets, or by phone and email, so they have a personal relationship and accountability to the people who eat their products. A farm with an open-door policy that welcomes visitors, invites press, and participates in its community is a farm that is likely doing things right and deserves your support.

To be healthy, eat meat, nose to tail, of all different types, harvested by hand or by someone you know.

RESOURCES

The American Meat Institute, "The United States Meat Industry at a Glance." Retrieved from www.meatami.com/ht/d/sp/i/47465/pid/47465.

Ben-Dor, M., A. Gopher, I. Hershkovitz, and R. Barkai, "Man the Fat Hunter: The Demise of *Homo erectus* and the Emergence of a New Hominin Lineage in the Middle Pleistocene (ca. 400 kyr) Levant." *PLoS ONE* 6, no. 12 (2001): e28689, doi:10.1371/journal.pone.0028689.

Kious, Brent M., "Hunter-Gatherer Nutrition and Its Implications for Modern Societies." *Nutrition Noteworthy* 5, no. 1 (2002). Retrieved from http://escholarship.org/uc/item/4wc9g8g4.

Masterjohn, Chris, "The Truth about the China Study." Retrieved from www.cholesterol-and-health.com/China-Study.html.

Reinhard, K.J., J. R. Ambler, and C. R. Szuter, "Hunter-Gatherer Use of Small Animal Food Resources: Coprolite Evidence." *International Journal of Osteoarchaeology* 17, no. 4 (2007): 416–28, doi 10.1002/oa.883.

Santarelli, R.L., F. Pierre, and D. E. Corpet, "Processed Meat and Colorectal Cancer: A Review of Epidemiologic and Experimental Evidence." *Nutrition and Cancer* 60, no. 2 (2008): 131–44, doi: 10.1080/01635580701684872.

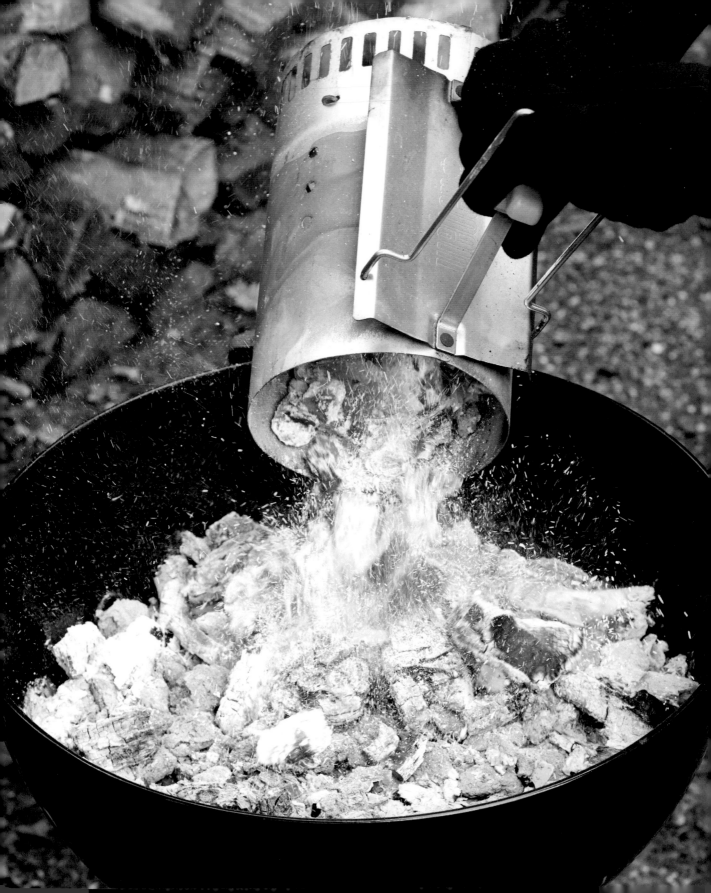

GETTING STARTED

"I grill, therefore I am." —**ALTON BROWN**

Selecting the right grill is the first step in getting started. There are big grills, little grills, grills loaded with gadgets, and others that are no frills and focused solely on grilling. To help you make the right choice, we're going to break down the three main types of grills—charcoal, gas, and electric—and give you our recommendations for which ones are the best for Paleo grilling.

CHARCOAL GRILLS

Charcoal grills are the grilling purist's first choice and are also our top pick for Paleo grilling. With charcoal, it's just you, the meat, and fire, an elemental battle that, if properly navigated, will result in an awesomely delicious meal. Charcoal has been used for cooking since the first primitive chefs huddled over their campfires with nothing more than a dead animal and a burning pile of wood, and for the modern caveman, the pleasures of charcoal cooking are just as primal.

Charcoal simply gives your food a flavor that can't be found anywhere else, and if you want your food to have that quintessential charred smoky taste, that signature of summertime, then you need to cook with coal. Coal also allows gives you the ability to crank up the heat. The more coals you pile up, the hotter the grill gets; there is no dial to hold you back. There are no limitations when it comes to cooking space, either; you can cook on the entire grill surface by spreading the coals around and you don't have to just stick to spots with burners.

On the downside, charcoal grills are definitely less convenient in that they require more cleanup, but this is Paleo grilling, so don't be afraid to get your hands dirty! Also, the fact that you are actually burning charcoal means that you cannot use these grills indoors; otherwise, you run the risk of carbon monoxide poisoning. The good news is that this forces you to get outside, another Paleo win!

BARBECUING OR GRILLING

Although the two terms are often used interchangeably, grilling and barbecuing are two distinct cooking methods. Grilling is what you do with burgers, steaks, and other foods that need direct, high heat. Barbecuing, on the other hand, uses indirect heat and smoke to cook tough cuts of meat, such as brisket and pork shoulder, over a long period of time. It can get confusing because some pieces of equipment, such as the Big Green Egg, allow you to either grill or barbecue your food, but if you're going to be a true Paleo grilling aficionado, it pays to know your lingo and cooking technique.

Briquettes versus Lumps

Briquettes are the processed food of grilling fuels. A typical briquette is a compressed lump of wood by-products and additives such as borax, peanut husks (called "chaff"), wax, and sodium nitrate. Most of the chemicals are probably burned away by the time the briquette is ready to cook with, but I'd rather not take my chances. If we're trying to do things the right way, we want to use only the best ingredients right from the start, which leads us to lump charcoal.

Lump charcoal is produced by burning hardwoods such as oak, cherry, and apple in the absence of oxygen. The result is a block of carbon and ash with no added chemicals, so your food will get only the pure sweet smoke and white-hot heat from the coals, exactly what we want for Paleo grilling. The downside is that lump charcoal is more difficult to light than briquettes are. We don't want to go through the trouble of sourcing better quality coal only to dump lighter fluid on it, so this means using a chimney starter. Chimney starters look like a metal pitcher with holes in the bottom and they are a cheap and easy way to get your coals ready quickly without the use of chemical accelerants such as lighter fluid.

As a bonus, the leftover ash from lump coal can be used as fertilizer for plants. Simply allow the spent coals to cool for at least 48 hours (or speed the process by pouring water on the coals and gently stirring) and then spread the ash over flower or vegetable beds. Ash contains potash, a water-soluble form of potassium, which is an important nutrient for plants.

Which Style of Charcoal Grill to Choose

The classic charcoal grill is the kettle-style grill made popular by the Weber company. Cheap, simple, and durable, this grill is a great starting point for the novice cook. You can do just about anything with it and it won't break the bank. These grills typically have an adjustable air valve on the lid, which allows you to control the amount of heat held inside the grill while cooking. The shape of the grill tends to hold in heat, however, so they aren't the best choice for barbecuing and smoking.

The low-end kettle grill models also tend to lack any built-in workspace for setting down ingredients, plates of meat, and tools, which may be inconvenient if you're cooking for a crowd, or if you don't have three hands. Premium kettle grills are available, and these do have amenities, such as built-in workspace, that make them an attractive choice. For all the tailgaters out there, there are portable kettle grills that are small enough to tend with one hand while sitting in your favorite folding chair.

"Egg-style" grills, such as the Big Green Egg and Broil King Steel Keg, are considerably more expensive than the kettle grills, but their price might be warranted by their increased durability and function. They can be used just like a standard grill, but the fact that they are built from materials that hold heat exceptionally well means that they are a great choice for barbecuing meats that need to be treated gently with low and slow heat.

Open grills, like the type often provided for community use at parks and recreational areas, lack lids and are therefore grills in the purest sense. You could technically prop a metal grate over a burned-out campfire and have an impromptu burger session with little muss or fuss. Higher end models of open grills do offer some amenities such as adjustable racks or rotisserie spits, allowing for better control over temperature and cooking technique.

Barrel grills, named for the fact that they were often made from leftover oil barrels (cleaned out, I hope!), are an excellent choice because they are often very affordable (some models are less than $100), offer a large amount of cooking space for feeding hungry crowds, and are just as well suited for barbecuing as they are for grilling. Larger models, often advertised as "competition smokers," can be big enough to smoke a whole hog and include attached fireboxes, specialized compartments for burning smoking wood.

SHOULD I BUY GLASS OR PLASTIC BOTTLES?

Plastic bottles typically contain a chemical called BPA, which is used to make the plastic softer and more pliable. Unfortunately for us, however, BPA in containers also leaches into the products inside, eventually making it into our bodies. In the human body, BPA disrupts hormones and can cause brain and reproductive issues. Buying products in glass bottles avoids this issue.

STARTING COALS WITH A CHIMNEY STARTER

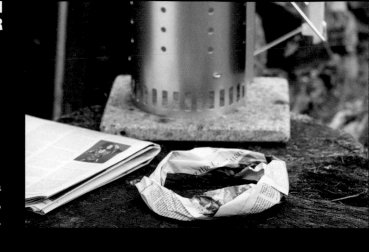

Roll a full sheet of newspaper into a tube and bring the ends together, forming a doughnut shape.

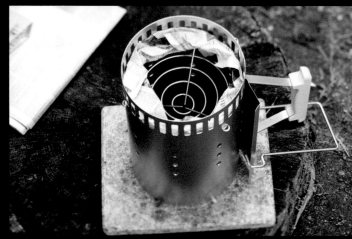

Turn the chimney starter over and put the rolled-up newspaper into the bottom of the starter.

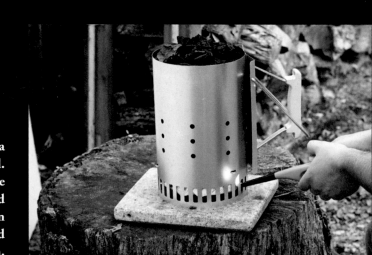

Put the starter right side up on a fire-safe surface and fill with charcoal. The bottom grate of your grill, the one that holds the coals, is recommended for this. Light the newspaper in several places with a long-stemmed grill lighter or wooden match.

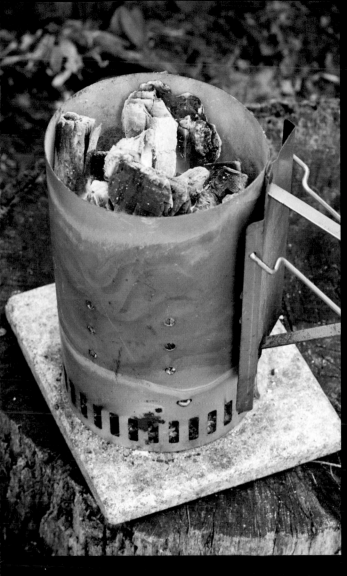

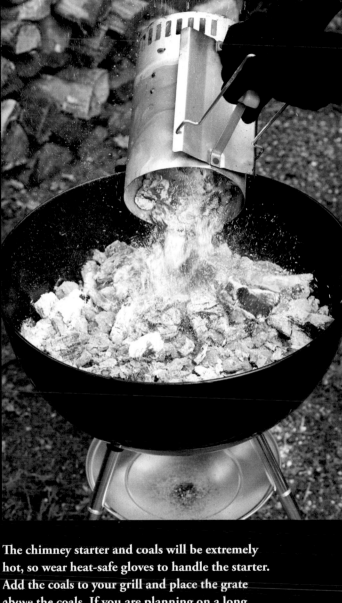

After the coals light, it will take approximately 20 minutes before they are ready. Depending on your particular chimney starter and coals, this time may vary, so watch for an orange glow coming up from the bottom of the starter with some of the top coals just starting to ash over; this will let you know that they are ready.

The chimney starter and coals will be extremely hot, so wear heat-safe gloves to handle the starter. Add the coals to your grill and place the grate above the coals. If you are planning on a long grilling session, you can start another chimney full of charcoal right away, adding more coals as needed to keep the temperature in range. *Warning:* The chimney starter itself is very hot and will remain so for quite a while. Place it on

GAS GRILLS

Although gas grills lack in the fire and flavor departments, they do have their benefits, which makes them a suitable second choice for Paleo grilling. Fueled by a tank of propane that lasts for many hours of grilling, a gas grill can be quickly fired up, making it a great option for someone who wants to grill on a regular basis. There is no reason to start an entire bag of charcoal when you want burgers for two! Precise control of temperature, a simple matter of turning a dial, also takes out much of the guesswork involved in charcoal grilling.

Gas grills can also be augmented by the addition of fireboxes that burn wood, imparting some of the smoky flavor associated with charcoal grilling. Some also have burners that you can use to prepare sauces and dual heat zones for direct- as well as indirect-heat grilling. Economy also favors gas grilling because refilling a tank is much cheaper, and easier to store, than buying multiple bags of quality charcoal.

When in doubt, follow the manufacturer's instructions for lighting and cooking with your gas grill.

ELECTRIC GRILLS

Electric grills are good for two things—college students and grill marks. Aside from that, they are little more that waffle irons for meat. This doesn't mean that they aren't useful (I've prepared many a hamburger on my trusty George Foreman), but that doesn't mean they are Paleo grilling approved. If you're stuck inside and have no other option, then go for electric, but don't call it grilling!

PREPARING YOUR GRILL

If you haven't used your grill for a while it might have a coating of gunk built up that you should remove before your next cookout. Start by getting the grill nice and hot for a good 15 to 20 minutes. This will burn off some of the old food and grease and will loosen up the rest, making it easier to clean. Once the food begins to loosen up, turn off the grill.

Use a stainless steel wire brush to clean the grates and burners. They may need to be removed and attacked with soap and water if vigorous brushing isn't doing the trick. Gas grills will also need to have their gas jets cleared out with a wire clothes hanger.

Clean out the inside of the grill, removing any charcoal residue and scraping down the sides and inside of the lid with a nylon paint scraper. Reassemble the grill. Using a paper towel, give the grates a thin coat of tallow to help keep food from sticking when you start grilling.

BLINGED-OUT GRILLS

The type of material your grilling surface is made of makes a big difference when it comes to cooking and cleanup. Porcelain-coated steel is okay, but I would avoid bent steel sheets because they are difficult to clean and don't heat evenly. Iron grills transfer heat well, but they are a pain to clean. A stainless steel grill is the best choice because it has good heat transfer and is easy to clean, but it's also the most expensive.

SMOKING WITHOUT A SMOKER

While a dedicated smoker, barrel, or egg-style grill designed for smoking (see page 27) is ideal for recipes that require tightly controlled temperatures and that perfect "thin blue smoke", you can still get good results on a standard grill. Assuming you have a common kettle style grill here are some guidelines to get you smoking.

1. Don't bother soaking your wood chips. The moisture will have to cook off before they start producing smoke anyway so it's an unnecessary step. All you have to do is wrap your chips in an aluminum foil pouch with a few slits cut into it to limit the rate of burning. You can then place the foil pouch directly over hot coals. Better yet, use wood chunks as these don't require any special preparation whatsoever.

2. Put your hot coals on only half of the bottom grill grate. On the other half, place an aluminum pan full of water. The water will help regulate the temperature in your grill as well as create steam that helps the meat retain moisture. If you have space, you can put an additional pan of water on the main grilling surface as well.

3. When positioning your main grilling grate, make sure that the hinged side is over your hot coals so you can easily refresh the coals or add additional wood chips/chunks during the cook.

4. The vents on your grill aren't just for show: properly using them makes a big difference. Crack the top vent (the exhaust damper) halfway and make sure it is positioned over the top of meat. This will create a convection current within the grill that draws smoke and heat over the food. The bottom vent (the intake damper) increases or decreases the amount of oxygen in the grill. Opening it wider increases the temperature by feeding the coals oxygen while closing it reduces the temperature. Just don't close it all the way or you will extinguish your coals!

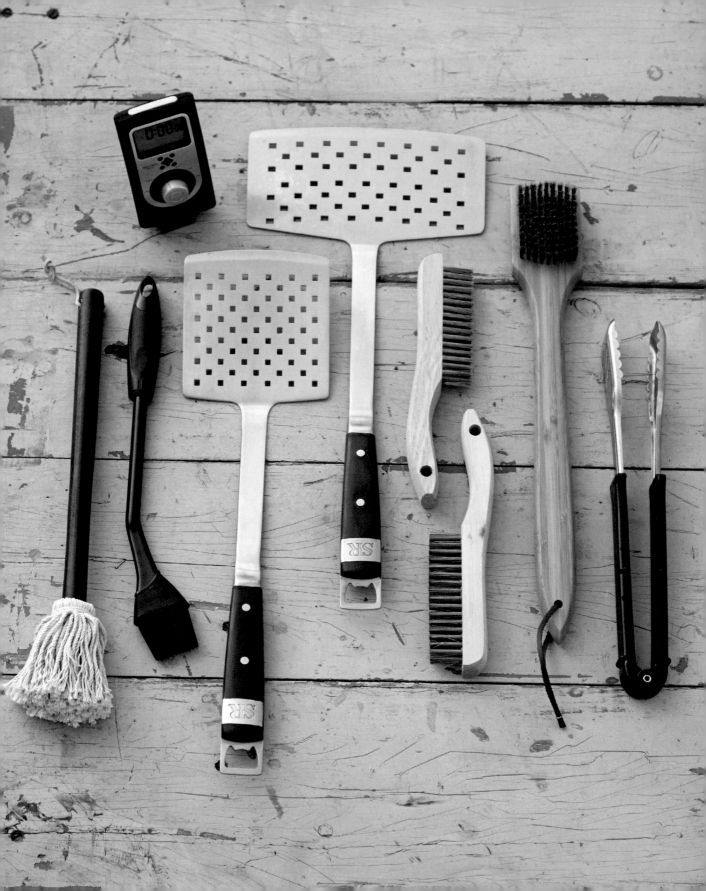

TOOLS FOR THE MODERN CAVEMAN

Although you can surely get by without too many gadgets, gizmos, or other grilling accessories, there are certain essential items that you might want to consider if you want to avoid burnt food, burnt fingers, and the other potential hazards that accompany cooking with fire.

GRILLING NECESSITIES

These are the tools we couldn't do without: They make grilling easier and the end product more delicious.

Temperature Gauge

Most grills come equipped with cheap temperature gauges that don't do a good job of telling you how hot your grill is, so you may want to invest in an upgraded model that will do a better job. However, even the best gauge is only a general indicator of the temperature inside your grill. **Recommendation:** Tel-Tru BBQ Smoker Thermometer (Teltru.com)

Meat Thermometer

Rare? Medium rare? Well done? Who knows? Well, you do if you have a meat thermometer. Despite the myth that you can judge doneness by pinching your hand and then pushing on your meat (no two hands are made alike and the same goes for different cuts of meat), an instant-read meat thermometer is the only way to get consistent results. The metal probe goes right into the meat of the matter (literally) to tell you exactly how done your dinner is. **Recommendation:** Thermoworks Splashproof Thermapen (Thermoworks.com)

Timer

Even if you don't have attention deficit disorder, it's easy to get distracted by all the different things you have to do to get a meal on the table. Setting a timer, whether it's a simple egg timer or even the alarm on your phone, can help avert disaster, or a visit from the fire department. **Recommendation:** Chef's Quad Timer by American Innovative (AmericanInnovative.com)

Grill Brush

Stainless steel or porcelain grates are easily scratched by traditional wire brushes, so go with a brass brush if you have either of these types. If you have a cast-iron or an expanded steel grate, a sturdy wire brush is what you'll need to scrub it clean before your next grilling session. **Recommendation:** Brass—Weber Brass Grill Brush (Weber.com), Wire—Forney Carbon Steel Wire Brush (ForneyInd.com)

Basting Brush

Basting, buttering, or brushing sauce onto your meat means that you'll need a brush that can hold onto liquids as well as hold up against heat. A silicone brush with fine, densely packed bristles offers both heat resistance and efficient sauce delivery. Boar's hair and nylon brushes are also known to shed, something you don't have to worry about with silicone.

Recommendation: Elizabeth Karmel's 15-inch (38 cm) Super Silicone Angled Barbecue Brush (ElizabethKarmel.com)

Sauce Mop

Even with a good basting brush, you might have trouble basting meat with thinner vinegar-based sauces. For these situations, keep a good cotton-threaded sauce mop handy.

Recommendation: Mr. Bar-B-Q 12-inch (30.5 cm) Barbecue Sauce Mop (MrBarBQ.com)

Tongs

Flipping burgers, maneuvering skewers, and manipulating grilled veggies with your bare hands could be considered an extreme sport, so save your skin and invest in a good set of barbecue tongs. Look for tongs that have a good grip (for your hand as well as scalloped edges for holding onto food), a solid tension mechanism, and the ability to lock when not in use.

Recommendation: Weber Style 6441 Professional-Grade Chef's Tongs (Weber.com)

Spatula

Getting food off of the grill and onto your plate can alternately require heavy lifting and a delicate touch. Go for a wide, sturdy spatula with a long, offset handle to make this balancing act a lot easier.

Recommendation: Steven Raichlen Stainless Steel Wide Spatula with Bottle Opener (BarbecueBible.com)

Chimney Starter

Starting several pounds of coals quickly, safely, and without any starter fluid is possible with a chimney starter. The design of a chimney starter allows air—and most important, oxygen—to flow, meaning that you'll be ready to grill in 15 minutes or less.

Recommendation: Weber 7416 Rapidfire Chimney Starter (Weber.com)

Grill Mitts

Grabbing a hot handle with a towel or a cotton oven mitt that happened to get wet could lead to some serious burns and would certainly put a damper on your day. Avoid the pain by investing in a good pair of grill mitts. Look for a mitt that comes almost up to your elbows (protect those arm hairs) and offers flexibility and dexterity as well as protection.

Recommendation: Steven Raichlen Best of Barbecue Extra Long Suede Gloves (BarbecueBible.com)

GRILLING SURFACES

Supplementing your grill's standard grate isn't necessary, but it does open up a wider range of cooking options, can save you from losing food to the hot coal god, and may even make your grilling healthier.

Griddle

Bacon on the grill. Need I say more? Throwing a griddle down makes meat candy available without having to walk back and forth into the kitchen. Of course, you can sauté vegetables on it too, if you're so inclined.

Grill Pan

Any seasoned grill master knows that, inevitably, food is going to fall through the grate, land on the coals, and become an inedible charred mess. A grill pan eliminates this concern because it allows heat to come through without your food doing the same.

ManGrate

Made from cast iron, the ManGrate holds tons of heat, making it perfect for leaving those signature grill marks on your steaks. It is also scalable, so you can buy more or less depending on the size of your grilling surface. Another bonus is that its design directs grease and cooking juices away from hot coals, preventing flare-ups and sending delicious vapor back to your meat. (ManGrate.com)

Cedar Planks

Cedar planks are a sure-fire way to give your food (especially fish) a delicious smoky flavor with minimal effort. As with wooden skewers, you'll have to soak them in water (at least 1 hour) before using; otherwise, you'll be serving charcoal salmon to your guests.

Himalayan Salt Blocks

Season and sear all in one step with these massive slabs of salt. Be sure to select a block that is at least $1^1/_2$ to 2 inches (3.8 to 5.1 cm) thick and of high grade. Heat the block slowly (indirectly over coals or by using a low setting on your gas grill) and wait until it's at least 500°F (260°C) before putting your food on it. *Hint:* If you don't have a thermometer that can check this for you, sprinkling a few droplets of water on the salt block will also work. When they sputter and steam instantly, you know you are good to go. (AtTheMeadow.com)

USEFUL TOYS

Whether it is to avoid the embarrassment of an empty propane tank or to create the ultimate bacon weave, these toys are nonessential but useful.

Grill Press

A heavy metal grill press can weight down foods to help them cook more evenly (can you say "bacon weave"?) or can be heated up directly to help cook and sear foods from two sides at the same time.

Smoker Box

A smoker box is simply a metal container with holes in it, so you can technically make one yourself by putting soaked wood chips into a foil pan, covering it with more foil, and then punching a few holes in the top. Purchasing a smoker box won't break the bank, though. If you plan on infusing your food with the delicious taste of smoke, then you might as well splurge.

Grill Light

Unless you only grill during the day, or under the light of a full moon (which would be super Paleo, by the way), you'll occasionally need some supplemental light to see what's going on inside your grill. A simple LED light that you can clip onto your grill's handle will do just fine for this job.

Propane Gas Monitor Gauge

Your friends are over, the steaks are on their way, and, tragically, you run out of gas. This isn't a concern for charcoal grillers, but for gas guys, a propane gas monitor gauge that attaches between your gas line regulator and propane cylinder will warn you when it's time to refill.

BASIC KITCHEN GEAR

Behind every great grilling session is a lot of behind-the-scenes prep work. Veggies need to be chopped, sauces need to be stirred, and meats need to be marinated. To ensure that you have everything you need to keep your prep kitchen running smoothly, here's a checklist of items that every grillmaster should have on hand.

- **Cutting board** (separate one for raw meat and another for other foods)
- **Knife set**—chef's knife, serrated knife, boning knife, paring knife, kitchen shears, and sharpening tool
- **Pots and pans**—heat-safe sauté pan, saucepot, stockpot
- **Colander** (strainer)
- **Cast-iron skillet**
- **Food processor**
- **Citrus reamer**
- **Vegetable peeler**
- **Zester**
- **Mortar and pestle**
- **Meat grinder** (or stand mixer attachment)
- **Piping bag** (or stand mixer sausage-making mixer attachment)
- **Blender**
- **Mixing bowl and whisk**
- **Ice cream maker**
- **Twine**
- **Mandoline**
- **Skewers** (metal and wooden)
- **Foil**
- **Disposable pans**

THE PRIMAL PANTRY

Keeping your kitchen stocked with plenty of Paleo-friendly foods means that you'll only really need to worry about tracking down main ingredients when you need to whip up a meal for two or a cookout for twenty. The initial "investment" at the grocery store might seem a little overwhelming, but over time, having a well-stocked pantry will pay off in better health for you and your family.

PALEO GRILLING STAPLES

This is a comprehensive list of the ingredients featured in *Paleo Grilling,* but don't sweat it if you can't track down everything. Feel free to exercise creativity in the kitchen, experiment with flavors, and substitute with similar ingredients when necessary.

Eggs

For freshness, you can't beat local. Try to find eggs from chickens raised on pasture where they have access to a wide variety of foods, from grass to crickets.

Fruits

Citrus (lemons, limes, oranges), berries (blueberries, strawberries, raspberries, blackberries), bananas, pears, cherries, tomatoes, and avocados

Vegetables

Cabbage, celery, garlic, onions, shallots, peppers (bell pepper, jalapeño, serrano, poblano, piquillo), ginger root, and mushrooms (technically a fungus, but they are sold in the vegetable section)

Nuts

Whole nuts (almonds, pine nuts, pecans, hazelnuts, pistachios, walnuts), nut butters (sesame seed tahini, cashew butter, almond butter, coconut butter), and nut flours (almond flour, coconut flour)

Paleo-Friendly Beverages

Kombucha, mineral water, hard cider, red and white wine, and coffee

Pickled and Preserved Foods

Olives, kimchi, and sauerkraut

Cured Meats

Bacon, pancetta, serrano ham, and prosciutto

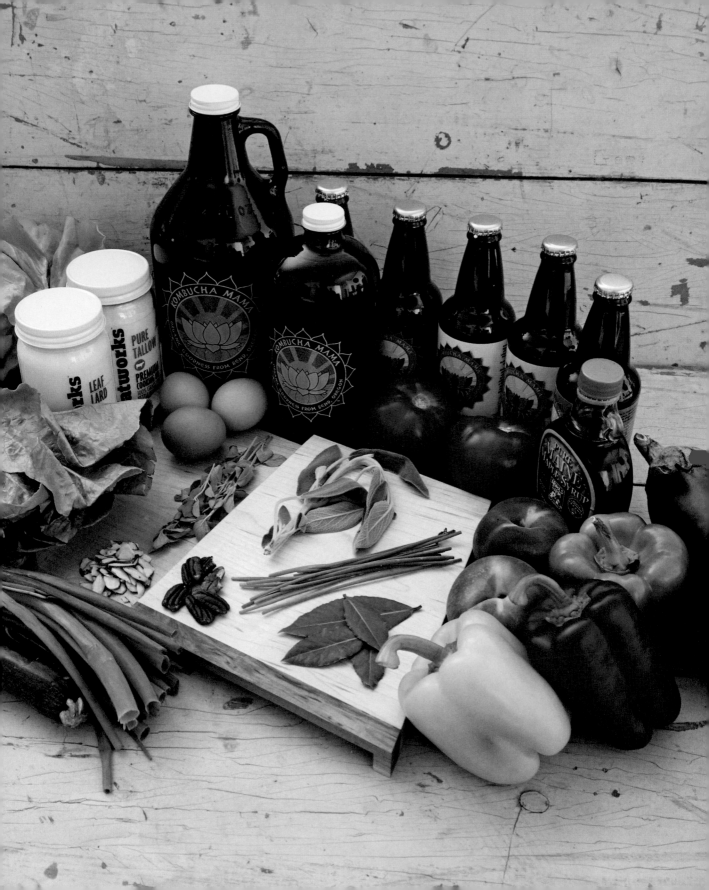

Canned Goods
Anchovies, full-fat coconut milk, and tomatoes (in BPA-free cans)

Stocks and Broths
Beef, veal, and chicken

Healthful Oils
Olive oil (light and extra virgin), lard (rendered pig fat), tallow (rendered beef fat), coconut oil (extra virgin and refined for high-heat cooking), avocado oil, flaxseed oil, and macadamia nut oil

Fresh Herbs
Basil, rosemary, thyme, parsley, oregano, cilantro, dill, tarragon, chives, and mint

Dried Herbs
Basil, oregano, thyme, parsley, lavender, and saffron

Spices
Paprika (hot, smoked, sweet), cinnamon, onion (powdered, dried, granulated), garlic powder, celery seed, turmeric, cumin, pepper (black, white, cayenne, chipotle, red pepper flakes), mustard (seeds and powdered), bay leaves, caraway seeds, and coriander

Salt
Sea salt, smoked salt, celery salt, kosher salt, and Himalayan sea salt

Condiments
Hot sauce, mustard (yellow, Dijon, coarse-ground "deli" style), coconut aminos, Worcestershire sauce, fish sauce, sriracha, and vinegars (white distilled vinegar, balsamic, Champagne vinegar, sherry, rice wine, apple cider vinegar, and red wine vinegar)

Unrefined Natural Sweeteners
Honey, coconut sugar, coconut nectar, and maple syrup

Miscellaneous Odds and Ends
Chocolate (dairy-free and soy-free), vanilla extract, and natural gut casings for sausage

MEAT CUTS

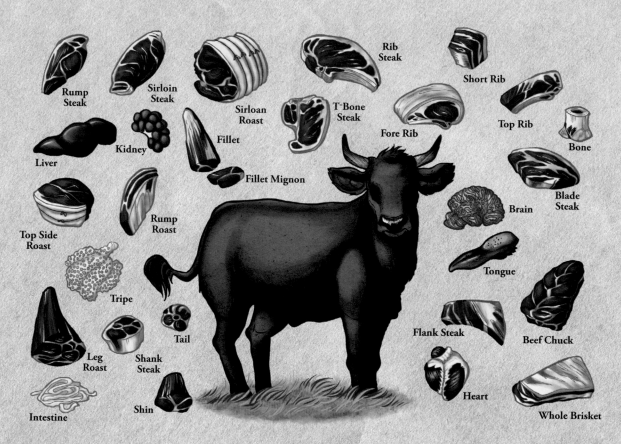

Rump Steak

Sirloin Steak

Sirloan Roast

Rib Steak

Short Rib

Liver

Kidney

Fillet

T-Bone Steak

Fore Rib

Top Rib

Bone

Fillet Mignon

Brain

Blade Steak

Top Side Roast

Rump Roast

Tongue

Tripe

Flank Steak

Beef Chuck

Leg Roast

Shank Steak

Tail

Heart

Whole Brisket

Intestine

Shin

BEEF

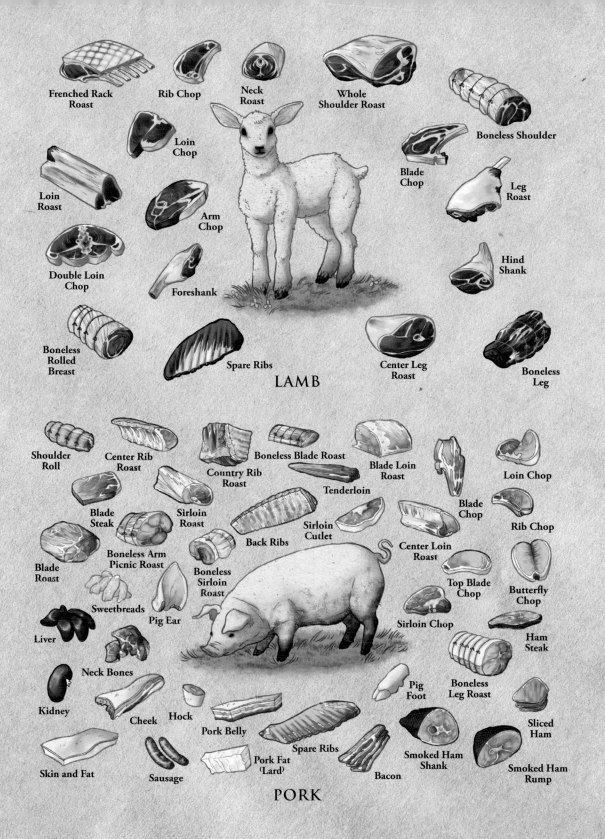

LAMB

Frenched Rack Roast
Rib Chop
Neck Roast
Whole Shoulder Roast
Boneless Shoulder
Loin Chop
Blade Chop
Leg Roast
Loin Roast
Arm Chop
Double Loin Chop
Foreshank
Hind Shank
Boneless Rolled Breast
Spare Ribs
Center Leg Roast
Boneless Leg

PORK

Shoulder Roll
Center Rib Roast
Boneless Blade Roast
Blade Loin Roast
Loin Chop
Country Rib Roast
Tenderloin
Blade Steak
Sirloin Roast
Sirloin Cutlet
Blade Chop
Rib Chop
Blade Roast
Boneless Arm Picnic Roast
Back Ribs
Center Loin Roast
Boneless Sirloin Roast
Top Blade Chop
Butterfly Chop
Sweetbreads
Pig Ear
Liver
Sirloin Chop
Ham Steak
Neck Bones
Pig Foot
Boneless Leg Roast
Kidney
Cheek
Hock
Pork Belly
Spare Ribs
Sliced Ham
Skin and Fat
Sausage
Pork Fat (Lard)
Bacon
Smoked Ham Shank
Smoked Ham Rump

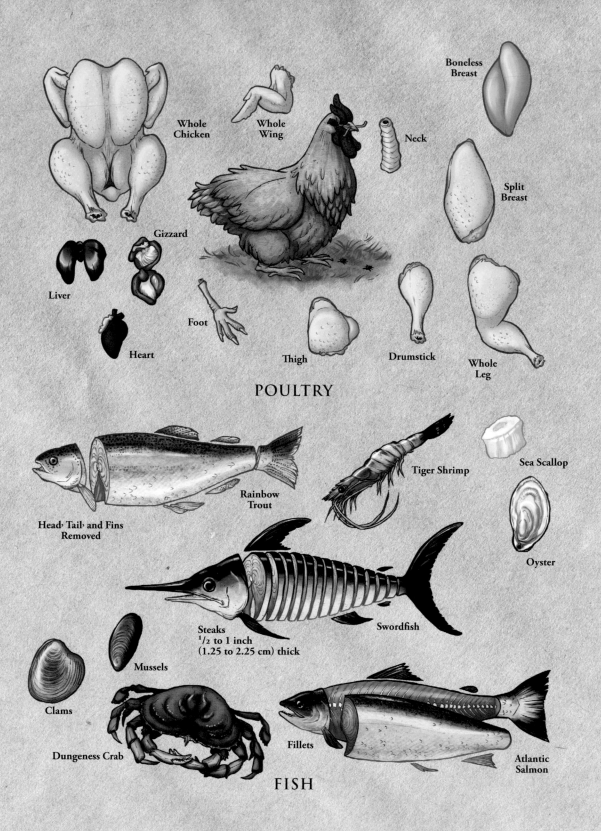

Whole
Chicken

Whole
Wing

Neck

Boneless
Breast

Split
Breast

Gizzard

Liver

Foot

Heart

Thigh

Drumstick

Whole
Leg

POULTRY

Rainbow
Trout

Tiger Shrimp

Sea Scallop

Head, Tail, and Fins
Removed

Oyster

Steaks
$^{1}/_{2}$ to 1 inch
(1.25 to 2.25 cm) thick

Swordfish

Mussels

Clams

Dungeness Crab

Fillets

Atlantic
Salmon

FISH

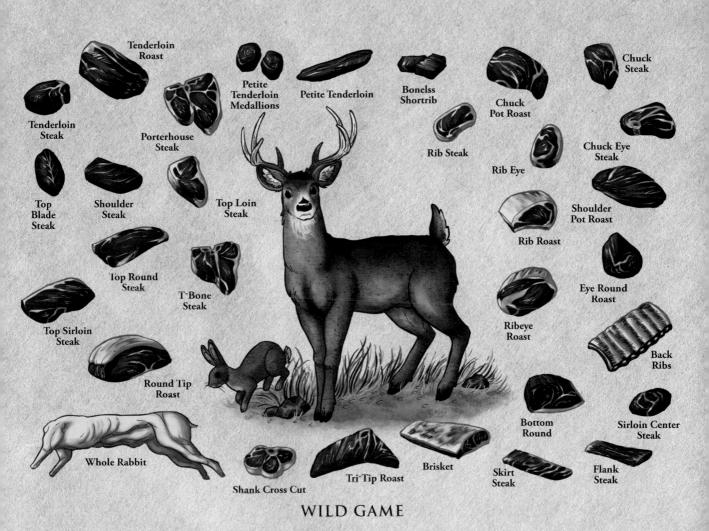

Tenderloin Roast

Petite Tenderloin Medallions

Petite Tenderloin

Bonelss Shortrib

Chuck Pot Roast

Chuck Steak

Tenderloin Steak

Porterhouse Steak

Rib Steak

Rib Eye

Chuck Eye Steak

Top Blade Steak

Shoulder Steak

Top Loin Steak

Rib Roast

Shoulder Pot Roast

Top Round Steak

T-Bone Steak

Ribeye Roast

Eye Round Roast

Top Sirloin Steak

Round Tip Roast

Back Ribs

Whole Rabbit

Shank Cross Cut

Tri-Tip Roast

Brisket

Skirt Steak

Bottom Round

Flank Steak

Sirloin Center Steak

WILD GAME

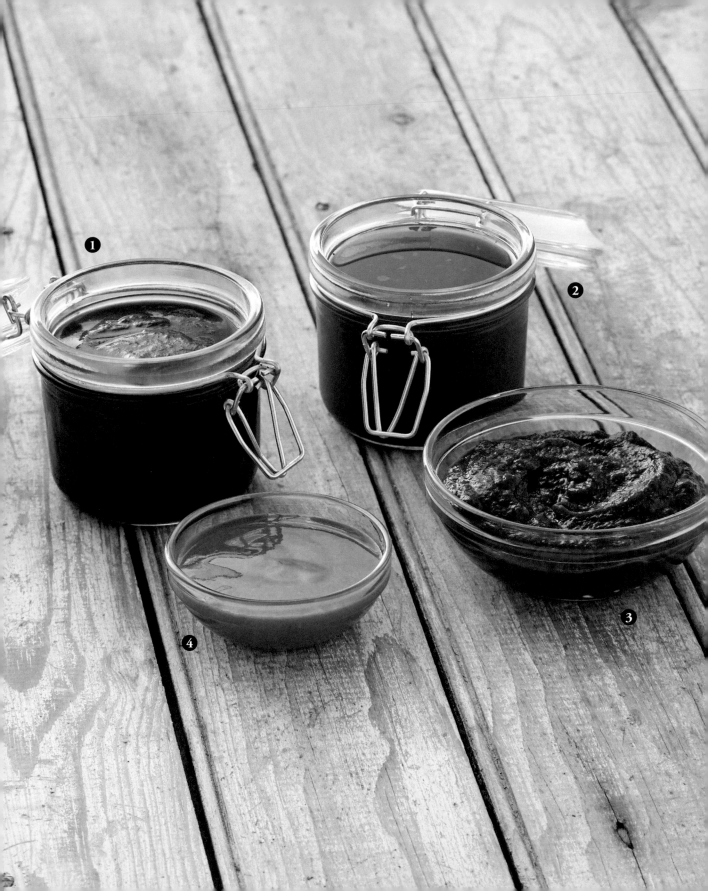

SAUCES RUBS AND MARINADES

CAVEMAN 'CUE (1)

$1/4$ cup (60 ml) freshly
squeezed orange juice

2 ounces (56 g)
minced red onion

1 cup (240 g)
Kicked-Up Ketchup (page 46)

1 teaspoon dark
chili powder

$1/2$ teaspoon smoked
sea salt

$1/2$ teaspoon
dried thyme

Heat the orange juice and
onions over medium heat
until it comes to a simmer.
Turn off the heat and add all
the other ingredients. Whisk
the barbecue sauce and cool
in the refrigerator.

YIELD: 1 CUP (240 G)

TANGY VINEGAR MOPPIN' SAUCE (2)

2 cups (470 ml)
apple cider vinegar

1 tablespoon (3.6 g) crushed
red pepper flakes

1 tablespoon (10 g)
minced garlic

$1 1/2$ teaspoons sea salt

1 tablespoon (6 g) freshly
ground black pepper

In a medium saucepan,
bring all the ingredients
to a boil over high heat.
Lower the heat and simmer
for 10 minutes. Turn the
heat off and allow to come
to room temperature.

YIELD: 2 CUPS (470 ML)

SWEET HEAT (3)

$1 1/2$ cups (300 g) packed
coconut sugar

$1 1/4$ cups (300 g) Kicked-Up
Ketchup (page 46)

$1/2$ cup (120 ml)
apple cider vinegar

$1/2$ cup (120 ml) water

1 teaspoon
cayenne pepper

1 teaspoon
chipotle pepper

Sea salt and freshly
ground black pepper,
to taste

Combine the coconut sugar,
ketchup, apple cider vinegar,
water, cayenne, and chipotle
pepper over medium heat.
Bring the sauce to a boil,
then reduce the heat and
simmer for 5 minutes.
Season with sea salt and
black pepper to taste.

YIELD: $3^1/_2$ CUPS (840 G)

HONEY MUSTARD (4)

1 cup (176 g)
yellow mustard

$2/3$ cup (230 g) honey

$1/3$ cup (67 g)
coconut sugar

$1/4$ cup (60 ml)
apple cider vinegar

2 teaspoons (3.6 g)
onion powder

Over medium heat, stir in
all the ingredients. Bring
the sauce to a boil and then
let it simmer for 5 minutes.

YIELD: 2 CUPS (350 G)

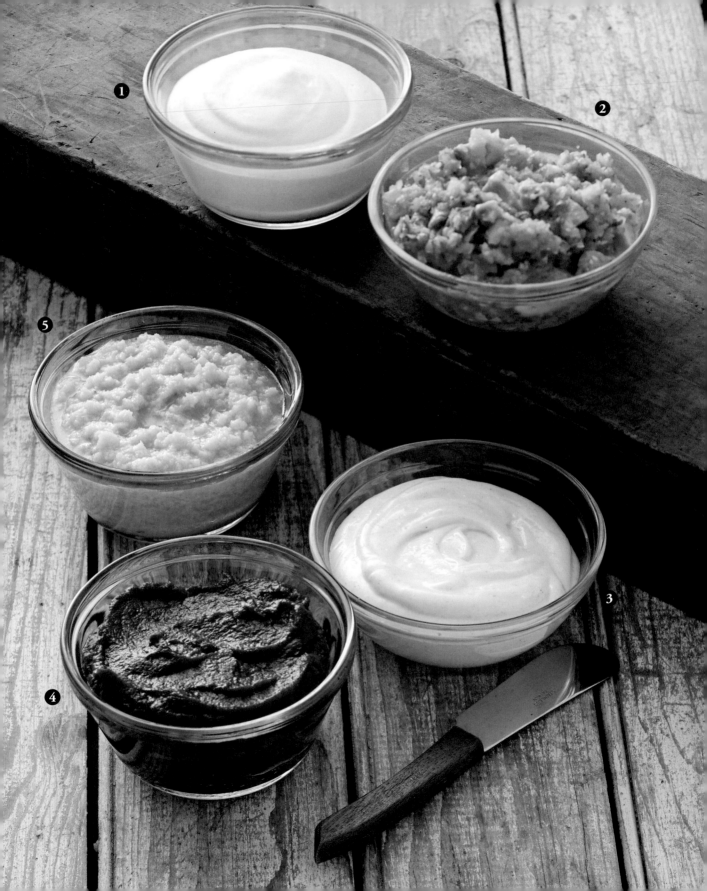

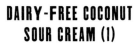

DAIRY-FREE COCONUT SOUR CREAM (1)

1 can (14 ounces, or 425 ml) full-fat coconut milk, chilled

1 tablespoon (15 ml) white vinegar

Open can of coconut milk and scoop out the hardened coconut cream on the top. Mix coconut cream and vinegar together until soft peaks form. Store in an airtight container in the refrigerator until ready to use.

YIELD: 1 CUP (240 G)

CHARRED TOMATILLO SALSA (2)

$^1/_2$ pound (228 g) tomatillos, husked, rinsed, and patted dry

$^1/_2$ large white onion, cut into 8 wedges

1 serrano chile, halved and seeded

3 tablespoons (45 ml) fresh lime juice

1 avocado, peeled and diced

2 tablespoons (2 g) chopped fresh cilantro

Sea salt

Preheat the grill. Grill the tomatillos, onion, and serrano until blistered, 12 to 15 minutes, turning halfway through. Let cool. Transfer the tomatillo mixture to a blender, add the lime juice, and pulse until a chunky puree forms. Fold in the diced avocado and cilantro and season with salt to taste.

YIELD: 2 CUPS (560 G)

PALEO MAYO (3)

1 clove garlic

2 chicken egg yolks or 1 duck egg yolk

Juice of 1 lemon

$^1/_2$ cup (120 ml) avocado or extra virgin olive oil

1 cup (235 ml) light olive oil

2 dashes of hot sauce

$^1/_2$ teaspoon white pepper

Pulverize the garlic with a mortar and pestle. Add the garlic, egg yolks, and lemon juice to a food processor and blend at medium speed (you could also use a blender for this, or even a bowl and whisk). Slowly drizzle a thin stream of the avocado or extra virgin olive oil into the mix, being careful not to add too much.

Finish by seasoning with hot sauce and white pepper. Seal the mayo in a clean container and refrigerate until ready to use. It will remain fresh for about a week.

YIELD: 1$^1/_2$ CUPS (375 G)

KICKED-UP KETCHUP (4)

16 ounces (454 g) tomato paste

1 tablespoon (7 g) onion powder

$^1/_2$ teaspoon cayenne pepper

1 teaspoon brown coconut sugar

1 teaspoon dry mustard

$^1/_3$ teaspoon ground allspice

$^1/_3$ teaspoon ground cloves

1 teaspoon cinnamon

1 cup (235 ml) apple cider vinegar

2 teaspoons (10 ml) Worcestershire sauce

Finely ground sea salt (to taste)

Combine all the ingredients except the salt together in a bowl and mix thoroughly. Add salt a little bit at a time, mixing between, to ensure the right amount. Store in an airtight jar in the refrigerator for up to a week.

YIELD: 2 CUPS (454 G)

AJO BLANCO (5)

8 cloves garlic, peeled

5 ounces (140 g) blanched almonds (the skinless kind you'll find in the baking aisle of the store)

Juice of 1 lemon

$^1/_2$ cup (120 ml) extra virgin olive oil

Place the cloves of garlic into a colander and then put the colander into a large pot of water. In a separate pot, prepare an ice bath. Bring the pot with the garlic to a boil. Once it has come to a boil, remove the garlic with the colander and plunge into the ice bath. Replace the water in the first pot and repeat the process two more times. This will mellow the garlic's flavor and make the resulting sauce less pungent.

Add the garlic and almonds to a food processor or blender and pulse several times, scraping down the sides with a spatula. Pulse three or four more times. Add the lemon juice and olive oil and blend. If it is too thick to blend properly, add 2 tablespoons (30 ml) cold water. Blend until slightly grainy.

YIELD: 1 CUP (260 G)

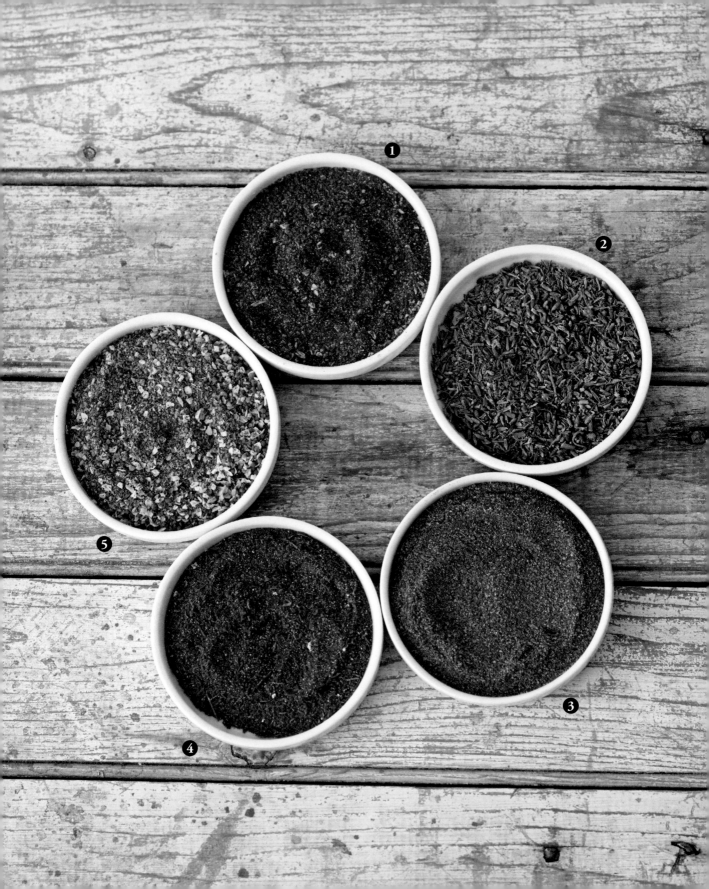

BEEF RUB (1)

3 tablespoons (21 g) hot paprika

3 tablespoons (54 g) coarse sea salt

2 tablespoons (30 ml) Worcestershire sauce

1 tablespoon (9 g) garlic powder

1 teaspoon cayenne

1 tablespoon (7 g) onion powder

1 tablespoon (6 g) freshly ground pepper

1 teaspoon cumin

Combine all the ingredients in a mixing bowl and mix thoroughly with a wire whisk. Store in a plastic container with an airtight lid.

YIELD: ³/₄ CUP (130 G)

CITRUS AND HERB SEAFOOD RUB (2)

1 tablespoon (3 g) dried thyme

1 tablespoon (3 g) dried lavender

1 tablespoon (2 g) dried basil

2 teaspoons (4 g) lemon zest

1 tablespoon (6 g) finely ground black pepper

1 teaspoon sea salt

5 tablespoons (75 ml) olive oil

Combine the dried herbs, lemon zest, black pepper, and salt. Mix it all together with a stiff whisk or fork. Add the olive oil and continue mixing into a paste.

YIELD: ¹/₂ CUP (100 G)

RIB RUB (3)

¹/₄ cup (28 g) sweet paprika

2 tablespoons (36 g) sea salt

2 tablespoons (15 g) smoked chile powder

2 tablespoons (12 g) ground black pepper

1 tablespoon (7 g) ground celery seed

2 tablespoons (18 g) dehydrated onion flakes

1 tablespoon (10 g) granulated garlic

2 tablespoons (4 g) rubbed sage

1 teaspoon dry mustard

¹/₂ cup (120 ml) coconut nectar

With a stiff whisk, stir together all of the ingredients in a mixing bowl until completely combined. Use almost immediately, as the rub will harden and be difficult to work with the longer it sits.

YIELD: 1 APPLICATION

WILD RUB (4)

1 teaspoon sweet paprika

¹/₂ teaspoon cayenne pepper

1 teaspoon cumin

1 teaspoon granulated garlic

¹/₂ teaspoon dried porcini powder

1 teaspoon dried thyme

1 teaspoon rubbed sage

1 teaspoon chili powder

¹/₂ teaspoon sea salt

Combine all of the ingredients in a mixing bowl and mix thoroughly. Store in a plastic container with an airtight lid.

YIELD: 2 TO 4 APPLICATIONS

PIG RUB (5)

4 tablespoons (44 g) coarsely ground mustard seed

4 tablespoons (24 g) coarsely ground black pepper

4 tablespoons (40 g) granulated garlic

1 tablespoon (5 g) cayenne pepper

2 teaspoons (6 g) dehydrated onion flakes

4 teaspoons (8 g) coconut sugar

Combine all the ingredients in a mixing bowl and mix thoroughly with a wire whisk. Store in a plastic container with an airtight lid.

YIELD: ³/₄ CUP (130 G)

POULTRY RUB
(NOT PICTURED)

2 tablespoon (14 g) paprika

1 tablespoon (10 g) granulated garlic

1 tablespoon (9 g) onion flakes

1 tablespoon (4 g) dried thyme

1 tablespoon (5.3 g) cayenne pepper

1 tablespoon (6 g) black pepper

1 tablespoon (3 g) dried oregano

1 tablespoon (2 g) dried basil

Combine all of the ingredients in a mixing bowl and mix together with a fork. Store in an airtight container.

YIELD: ¹/₂ CUP (54 G)

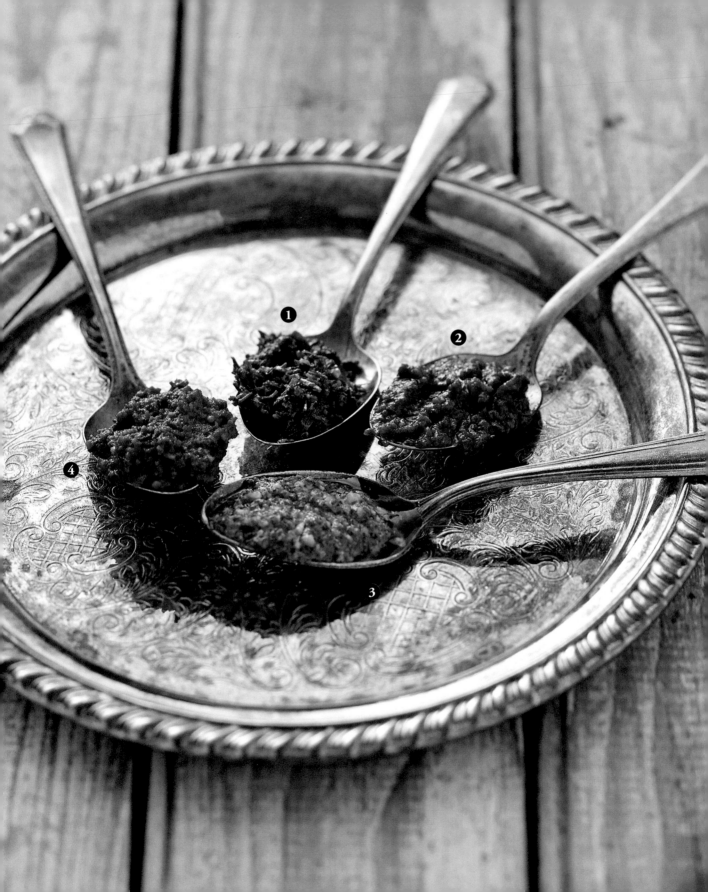

GREMOLATA (1)

THIS RECIPE COMES FROM MICHELLE NORRIS, CHEF CAVEWOMAN AT ECLECTIC KITCHEN EVOLVED.

1 cup (40 g) fresh basil
1 cup (28 g) fresh rosemary
1 cup (40 g) fresh thyme
1 cup (64 g) fresh oregano
4 cloves garlic, minced
$^1/_2$ teaspoon coarse sea salt
1 cup (235 ml) extra virgin olive oil

In a small mixing bowl, combine all of the ingredients. Using a fork, work everything together into a paste. Store for up to a week in an airtight container.

YIELD: 4 CUPS (400 G)

HARISSA (2)

9 ounces (252 g) long fresh chiles
1 tablespoon (7 g) caraway seed
1 tablespoon (7 g) cumin
1 teaspoon black cumin
4 cloves garlic
$3^1/_2$ ounces (100 g) piquillo peppers
1 tablespoon (15 g) tomato paste
1 tablespoon (15 ml) red wine vinegar
2 teaspoons (4 g) smoked paprika
6 tablespoons (90 ml) extra virgin olive oil, divided
Salt and pepper to taste

Combine all the ingredients in a food processor, reserving 1 tablespoon (15 ml) of olive oil. Blend until completely smooth, scraping the sides periodically. Pour into a container with an airtight lid. Top with the remaining olive oil to prevent oxidation.

YIELD: 1 CUP (225 G)

CHIMICHURRI (3)

6 cloves garlic
1 ounce (28 g) chopped white onion
2 bunches fresh parsley, washed, stemmed, and roughly chopped
4 tablespoons (16 g) chopped fresh oregano
$^1/_2$ cup (120 ml) olive oil
1 tablespoon (15 ml) lime juice
Sea salt
Red pepper flakes

Pulse the garlic and onion in a food processor until finely chopped. Add the parsley and oregano and pulse briefly. While pulsing, separately add the olive oil and lime juice in steady streams until fully incorporated. Do not puree, however, as chimichurri should have the consistency of a pesto. Season with salt and red pepper flakes to taste. Store in the refrigerator until ready to serve.

YIELD: ABOUT 1 CUP (240 G)

ROMESCO (4)

$^1/_4$ cup (60 ml) boiling water
2 teaspoons (2 g) saffron strands
4 dried ancho chile peppers
$3^1/_2$ ounces (100 g) blanched almonds
$1^3/_4$ ounces (50 g) hazelnuts
$5^1/_4$ ounces (150 g) piquillo peppers
1 to $1^1/_2$ tablespoons (15 to 22 ml) sherry vinegar
$^1/_2$ teaspoon smoked paprika
Sea salt and freshly ground black pepper to taste

Pour the boiling water into a ceramic container and add the saffron. Next, soak the ancho peppers in warm water to cover for 20 minutes. Remove the softened chiles from the water and discard the water. Break open the chiles and remove the seeds and stems. Cut the chiles into eighths and add to a food processor. Add all the remaining ingredients to the food processor, including the water used for steeping the saffron. Puree until almost smooth. Allow to cool completely and store in an airtight container.

YIELD: $^3/_4$ CUP (170 G)

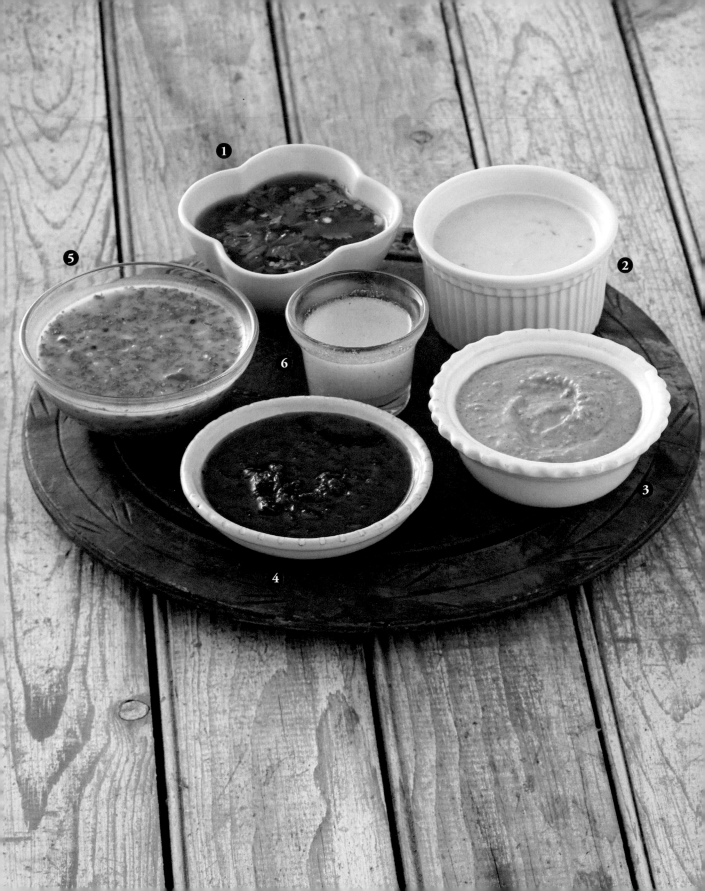

SOY-FREE SOY SAUCE–STYLE MEAT MARINADE (1)

$^1/_2$ cup (120 ml) coconut aminos

$^1/_2$ cup (120 ml) extra virgin olive oil

Juice of 2 limes

2 teaspoons (5 g) smoked paprika

6 large cloves garlic, minced

2 tablespoons (3 g) chopped fresh rosemary

2 tablespoons (5 g) chopped fresh thyme

2 tablespoons (12 g) coarsely ground black pepper

2 teaspoons (12 g) sea salt

Combine all the ingredients in a mixing bowl and whisk well until completely incorporated. Store in a container with a screw-on top, leaving about 1 inch (2.5 cm) of room at the top so that it can be shaken right before using. Refrigerate for up to 1 week.

YIELD: 1$^1/_4$ CUPS (295 ML)

WHITE BALSAMIC VINAIGRETTE (2)

$^1/_2$ cup (120 ml) extra virgin olive oil

$^1/_2$ cup (120 ml) white balsamic vinegar

1 clove garlic, crushed

1 teaspoon mustard powder

Pinch of salt

Ground black pepper to taste

In a small bowl, whisk together the olive oil, white balsamic vinegar, garlic, and mustard powder. Season to taste with salt and black pepper.

YIELD: 1 CUP (235 ML)

COCONUT RED CURRY SAUCE (3)

1 can (14 ounces, or 425 g) full-fat coconut milk

$^1/_4$ purple onion, chopped

1 stalk fresh lemongrass, minced

2 tablespoons (30 ml) sriracha sauce, or 1 or 2 fresh red chiles

1-inch (2.5 cm) piece fresh ginger root, peeled and sliced

1 teaspoon ground cumin

$^3/_4$ teaspoon ground coriander

$^1/_4$ teaspoon ground white pepper

2 tablespoons (30 ml) fish sauce
(Red Boat brand is great quality)

1 teaspoon coconut sugar

$1^1/_2$ tablespoons (11 g) chili powder

2 tablespoons (30 ml) freshly squeezed lime juice

Add all the ingredients to a food processor or blender and process until smooth.

YIELD: 2 CUPS (470 ML)

ASIAN PEAR BBQ MARINADE (4)

2 tablespoons (30 ml) sriracha hot Thai chili sauce

$^1/_4$ cup (60 ml) mirin (if you can't find mirin, substitute dry sherry or sweet Marsala cooking wine)

$^1/_2$ Asian pear, shredded

2 tablespoons (30 ml) sesame oil

2 tablespoons (40 g) honey

1 tablespoon (15 ml) fish sauce
(Nuoc Mam Vietnamese fish sauce is a good brand)

1 tablespoon (15 ml) coconut aminos

Combine all ingredients in a small bowl and whisk together until fully mixed.

YIELD: $^3/_4$ CUP (180 ML)

A WORD ABOUT HCAS

Potentially toxic compounds called heterocyclic amines (HCAs) are formed when meat is cooked over high heat, such as in grilling and smoking. However, marinades, especially those containing herbs and spices, dramatically reduce HCA formation. So marinate your meat and boost the healthfulness and flavor of your food!

ADOBO MARINADE (5)

½ cup (120 ml) lime juice
½ cup (120 ml) white wine vinegar
½ cup (120 ml) sesame oil
½ cup (120 ml) olive oil
2 tablespoons (12 g) finely ground black pepper
2 tablespoons (20 g) minced garlic
1 fresh jalapeño, diced
1 bunch fresh cilantro, chopped
1 bunch fresh curly parsley, chopped
1 tablespoon (4 g) red pepper flakes

Combine all the ingredients in a large mixing bowl and whisk until completely combined.

YIELD: 2 CUPS (470 ML)

SWEET AND SAVORY SPICE BRINE (6)

1 gallon (3.6 L) distilled water
4 cinnamon sticks
10 whole cloves
¼ cup (20 g) whole coriander
4 jalapeños, halved
1 ounce (28 g) fresh thyme sprigs
1 ounce (28 g) fresh rosemary sprigs
1 medium yellow onion, unpeeled, quartered
1 cup (340 g) honey
½ cup (288 g) sea salt
1 cup (235 ml) apple cider vinegar
2 apples, quartered

Combine all of the ingredients in a large stainless steel stockpot. Bring to a boil over high heat and then turn the heat to low. Let simmer for 5 minutes, and then turn off the heat. Let sit for 1 to 2 hours to allow the herbs and spices to infuse the brine and to cool to room temperature. Strain through a medium strainer into a large plastic container. Refrigerate overnight before using to brine meat.

YIELD: 1 GALLON (3.6 L)

"I hate people who are not serious about meals. It is so shallow of them."
—OSCAR WILDE, *The Importance of Being Earnest*

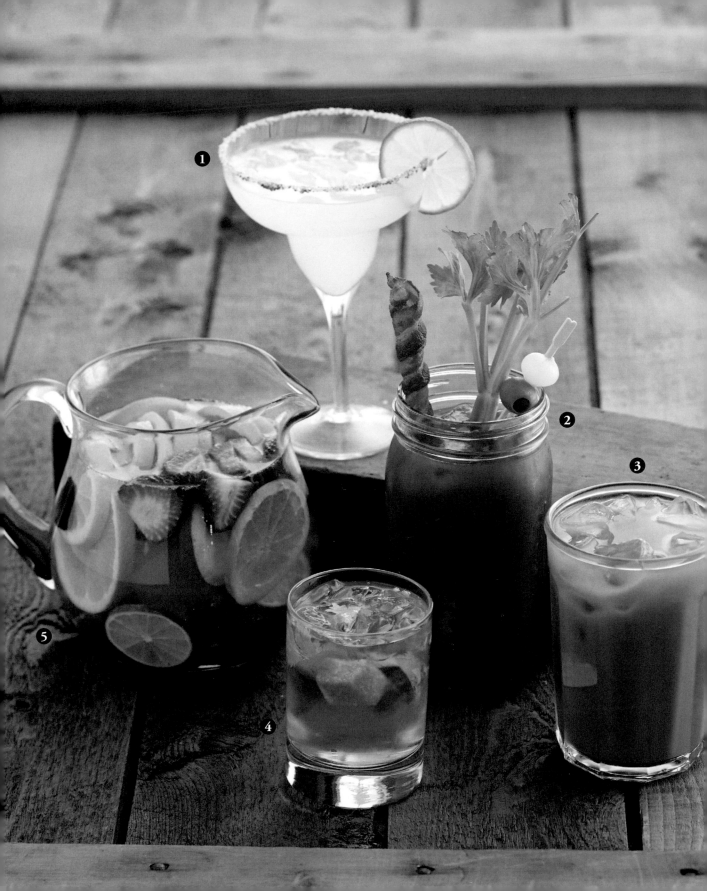

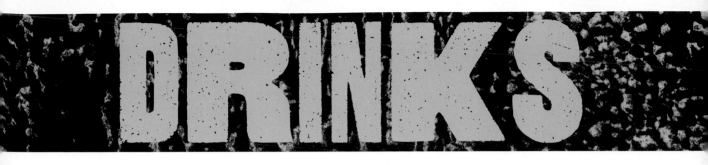

DRINKS

FOR VEGETABLE JUICE BASE:

1 can (28 ounces, or 784 g) whole peeled tomatoes

¹/₂ onion, chopped

2 cloves garlic

1 beet, chopped

1 carrot, chopped

1-inch (2.5 cm) horseradish root

2 small cucumbers, chopped

¹/₄ cup (15 g) fresh parsley

FOR BACON STRAWS:

4 strips bacon

Coconut nectar

FOR MIXER:

1 cup (235 ml) vodka

¹/₂ cup (120 ml) fresh lemon juice

3 tablespoons (45 ml) lime juice

1 tablespoon (15 ml) olive juice

¹/₂ teaspoon each celery salt, kosher salt, and garlic powder

¹/₄ teaspoon black pepper

1 dash each hot sauce and Worcestershire sauce

FOR GARNISH:

Green olives

Celery sticks

Pickled vegetables (page 64)

THE BLOODY CAVEMAN

TO MAKE THE JUICE BASE: Juice the fresh vegetables and parsley in a juicer, combine in a large pitcher, and refrigerate for 2 hours to chill.

TO PREPARE THE BACON STRAWS: Preheat the oven to 325ºF (170ºC, or gas mark 3). Roll sheets of aluminum foil into four 6- to 8-inch (15 to 20 cm) long pieces about the size of a pretzel rod. Wrap a piece of bacon in a spiral pattern around each piece of foil, ensuring that the edges overlap slightly. Brush the bacon straws with the coconut nectar and place on a wire rack on a baking sheet. Bake until crisp, 15 to 20 minutes. Remove from the oven and let cool on the wire rack. When the bacon has cooled, carefully remove the aluminum foil.

TO PREPARE THE MIXER: Add the mixer ingredients to the pitcher with the vegetable juice base. Stir to combine.

TO PREPARE THE GARNISH: Fill 4 tall glasses with ice and pour the Bloody Caveman mix over. Garnish with the olives, celery sticks, and pickled vegetables. Serve with a bacon straw.

YIELD: 4 SERVINGS

1. The Ultimate Paleorita (page 58)
2. The Bloody Caveman (page 57)
3. Cold-Brewed Cafe Con Leche (page 59)
4. Fruit and Herb Infused H$_2$O (page 59)
5. Mixed Berry Sangria (page 58)

THE ULTIMATE PALEORITA

FOR ORANGE LIQUEUR:

6 organic oranges

1 quart (1 L) brandy

FOR MARGARITAS:

$1^1/_2$ cups (355 ml) blanco tequila

$^3/_4$ cup (180 ml) orange liqueur

$^3/_4$ cup (180 ml) freshly squeezed lime juice

8 cups (2 L) crushed ice

FOR GARNISH:

2 tablespoons (36 g) sea salt

2 tablespoons (25 g) coconut sugar

6 lime wedges

TO PREPARE THE ORANGE LIQUEUR: Peel the rind of the oranges with a vegetable peeler. Remove any white pith, which will cause the final product to be bitter. Put the orange peels in a large mason jar and cover with the brandy. Seal the jar and let soak for 4 weeks. Strain the orange liqueur first with a wire strainer to remove the large pieces of peel. Strain the resulting liquid two more times through the wire strainer lined with a coffee filter (use a fresh filter each time) or until the liqueur is clear. Store the orange liqueur in a glass bottle in the refrigerator until ready to use.

TO PREPARE THE MARGARITAS: Combine the tequila, orange liqueur, lime juice, and ice in a pitcher.

TO PREPARE THE GARNISH: Mix together the sea salt and coconut sugar on a plate. Moisten the rim of your margarita glasses and dip the rims of the glasses halfway around into the sugar/salt mixture. Pour the margarita mix into the glasses and garnish with a wedge of lime.

YIELD: 6 SERVINGS

MIXED BERRY SANGRIA

1 bottle (1 L) white wine (such as a Riesling, Albarino, Chablis, Gewürztraminer, Pinot Gris, Chardonnay, or Sauvignon Blanc)

3 oranges, cut into wedges

1 lemon, cut into wedges

1 lime, cut into wedges

1 cup (170 g) sliced strawberries

1 cup (145 g) blueberries, fresh or frozen

1 cup (125 g) raspberries, fresh or frozen

2 cups (470 ml) carbonated mineral water (such as Topo Chico or Perrier)

Pour the wine into the pitcher and squeeze the juice wedges from the orange, lemon, and lime into the wine. Toss in the fruit wedges (leaving out seeds, if possible). Chill overnight. Add the remaining fruit and carbonated water just before serving.

YIELD: 4 SERVINGS

COLD-BREWED CAFE CON LECHE

1½ cups (180 g) coarsely
ground coffee beans

4 cups (946 ml) cold water

Full-fat coconut milk, almond milk,
or any other grain-free, soy-free,
dairy-free milk product, to taste

Ice

Ground cinnamon, for garnish

Add the ground coffee to a French press and mix thoroughly with the water. The coffee will tend to clump up, so stir it around a bit to make sure all of the grounds are immersed. Cover the top of the French press with plastic wrap or foil and let the coffee steep for 12 to 24 hours.

Using the French press filter, press the solids out of the coffee and pour the cold-brewed coffee into a sealable container. Place the coffee concentrate into your refrigerator to cool (at least 2 hours).

When you are ready to enjoy your cold-brewed coffee, mix with coconut or almond milk and pour over ice. It's also so smooth that you can enjoy it straight "on the rocks." Garnish with a dash of cinnamon and rock on.

YIELD: 4 SERVINGS

FRUIT- AND HERB-INFUSED H2O

FOR WATERMELON-CILANTRO:

2 cups (300 g) cubed fresh watermelon

2 cups (32 g) fresh cilantro

2 quarts (1.8 L) cold water

FOR LEMON-BASIL:

2 lemons, sliced

2 cups (80 g) fresh basil leaves

2 quarts (1.8 L) cold water

FOR PINEAPPLE-MINT:

2 cups (330 g) peeled and cubed fresh pineapple

2 cups (80 g) fresh mint leaves

2 quarts (1.8 L) cold water

Cover the fruit and herbs with the cold water. Allow the mixture to steep in the refrigerator for 2 to 3 hours before serving.

YIELD: 6 TO 8 SERVINGS

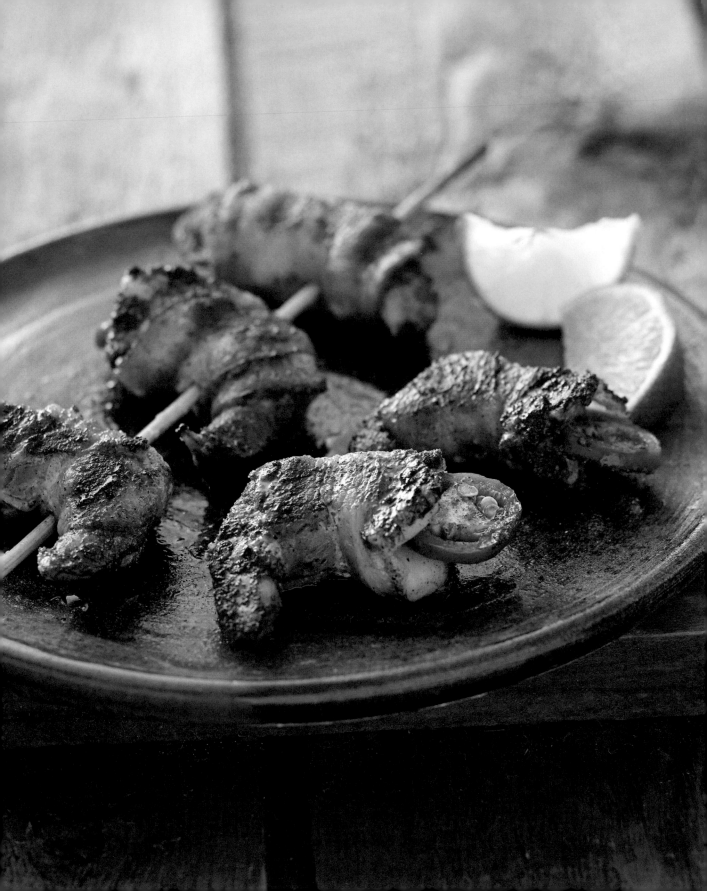

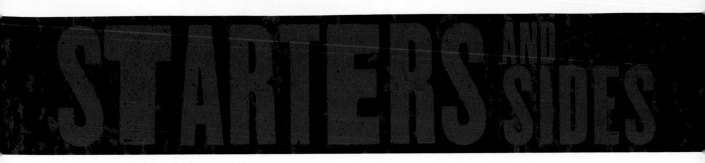
2 teaspoons (6 g) garlic powder

2 teaspoons (5 g) paprika

2 teaspoons (5 g) freshly
ground black pepper

$^1/_2$ teaspoon cayenne pepper

2 pounds (907 g) large shrimp,
peeled, deveined, and rinsed

3 jalapeños, cut in half, seeded,
and cut into thin slices

1 pound (454 g) bacon
strips, cut in half

$^1/_4$ cup (56 g)
coconut oil, melted

1 lime, quartered

POPPIN' SHRIMP

THE FLAVOR OF THIS DISH POPS WITH PLENTY OF SPICE AND
SALTY BACON.

Soak 8 wooden skewers in water to cover for 30 minutes (or use metal skewers).

In a small bowl mix together the garlic powder, paprika, black pepper, and cayenne pepper. Place the shrimp in a large bowl and season with three-fourths of the spice mixture, tossing to evenly coat.

Working with one shrimp at a time, make a slit about $^3/_4$ inch (2 cm) long at the base of the shrimp. Place 1 jalapeño slice in the slit, then wrap the base of the shrimp all the way around with half a slice of bacon. Repeat with the rest of the shrimp.

Thread the shrimp onto the skewers and season lightly with the remaining one-fourth spice mixture. Brush the shrimp lightly with coconut oil.

Preheat your grill to high heat. Grill the shrimp until the bacon crisps and the shrimp are just cooked through, 2 to 3 minutes per side. Remove to a platter and serve with the lime wedges.

YIELD: 8 SERVINGS

"The only time to eat diet food is while you're waiting for the steak to cook." —**JULIA CHILD**

12 eggs

$^1/_4$ cup (14 g) drained sun-dried tomatoes

1 small clove garlic, smashed

Pinch of cayenne pepper

$^1/_2$ cup (125 g) Paleo Mayo (page 47)

24 pieces pancetta ham, sliced into $^1/_4$-inch (6 mm)- thick rounds

Fresh basil leaves, rolled and thinly sliced (chiffonade)

Himalayan sea salt

DEVILED EGGS ARE PACKED WITH PROTEIN AND PLENTY OF HEALTHY FATS FROM EGG YOLKS. WE'VE SWAPPED MAYO OUT FOR A HOMEMADE TOMATO AIOLI. THE COMBINATION OF TOMATO, OLIVE OIL, AND BASIL WILL REMIND YOU OF BRUSCHETTA, BUT THE CRISPY PANCETTA WILL GIVE TEXTURE AND A SALTY CRUNCH TO EACH BITE.

Place the eggs in a large saucepan and cover with water. Heat over high until the water begins to boil. Cover the pan and turn the heat to low. Let the eggs cook for 1 minute. Turn the heat off, leaving the pot covered for an additional 14 minutes.

Alternatively, you could "hard bake" your eggs in the oven or even on the grill. To do this, simply preheat your oven or grill to 325°F (170°C, or gas mark 3) and place the eggs directly on the grill or oven grate (put a pan underneath them if you are using your oven in case they break). Let them cook for 30 minutes with the grill lid or oven door closed, and then carefully remove with tongs or oven mitts.

Once the eggs are cooked, chill them under cold running water. Once they are cool enough to handle, carefully crack the eggshells and remove. Return the eggs to a bowl of cold ice water to completely chill. Dry the eggs with a paper towel and slice in half lengthwise. Remove the yolks and put them in a large bowl and put the whites on a separate plate.

In a food processor, pulse the sun-dried tomatoes with the garlic and cayenne until finely chopped, then puree until smooth. Add the mayo and pulse just until blended.

Mash the egg yolks with a fork and mix with the sun-dried tomato mayonnaise until well combined. Spoon the filling into the egg white halves, using a pastry piping bag if you want to get fancy.

Preheat the oven to 400°F (200°C, or gas mark 6). Drape the slices of pancetta over the sections of 2 upside-down muffin tins, place each tin on a baking sheet, and bake for 10 to 12 minutes, until crispy. Allow the pancetta cups to cool before filling each cup with a deviled egg.

Garnish each cup with a few strands of basil and a small pinch of Himalayan salt.

YIELD: 24 SERVINGS

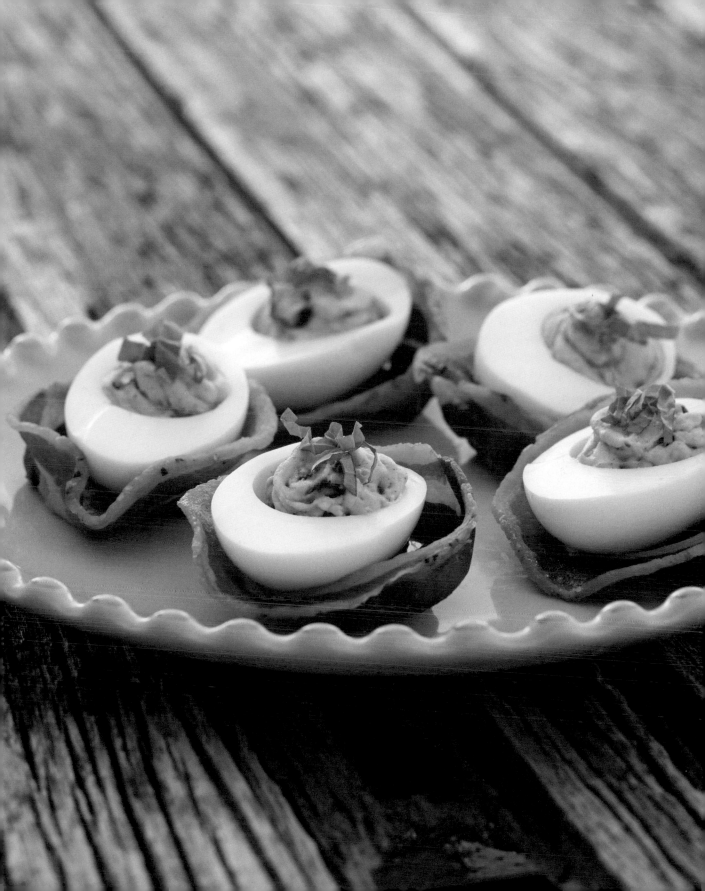

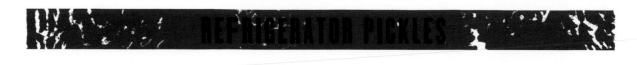

FOR BRINE (ENOUGH FOR APPROXIMATELY 1 POUND [454 G] OF VEGETABLES):

2 cups (470 ml) white vinegar

2 cups (470 ml) water

$^1/_2$ cup (100 g) coconut sugar

1 tablespoon (18 g) sea salt

6 whole cloves garlic

1 tablespoon (5 g) whole peppercorns

1 tablespoon (11 g) whole mustard seed

Pinch of red pepper flakes

1 bunch fresh dill, roughly chopped

FOR PICKLES:

$^1/_2$ pound (227 g) fresh green beans, ends and strings removed

2 large carrots, peeled and cut into 4- or 5-inch (10 or 12.5 cm) sticks (cut the carrot in half, then divide each half twice more)

8 stalks asparagus (green or white)

2 red bell peppers, cored, seeded and cut into $^1/_2$-inch (1.3 cm)-thick sticks

QUICK PICKLING LEAVES VEGETABLES CRUNCHY AND BRIGHTLY FLAVORED. IT IS A PERFECT WAY TO PRESERVE GARDEN-FRESH VEGETABLES, AND PICKLES ARE A NATURAL COMPLEMENT TO GRILLED MEATS, A GREAT ADDITION TO SALADS, OR A TANGY STAND-ALONE SNACK.

TO PREPARE THE BRINE: Heat the vinegar, water, sugar, and salt in a saucepan over medium heat. Bring the mixture to a boil and then lower the heat, stirring to ensure that all the solids are dissolved. Allow the brine to cool before adding the garlic, peppercorns, mustard seed, red pepper flakes, and dill.

TO MAKE THE PICKLES: Bring a large pot of salted water to a boil over high heat and prepare an ice water bath. Blanch the green beans, carrots, asparagus, and bell peppers in the boiling water, quickly remove with a slotted spoon, and cool in the ice bath for 60 seconds to halt the cooking.

Pack the vegetables into a quart (940 ml) mason jar and cover with the brine. Store the jar in the refrigerator for 12 to 24 hours before serving.

YIELD: 1 QUART (940 ML)

WHAT ELSE CAN I PICKLE?

I hesitate to say that you can pickle *anything*, but you can definitely pickle a lot, with good results. Leftover watermelon rind is great pickled, as are hard-boiled and peeled quail eggs. Get creative and brine something good today!

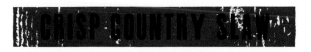 

PRE-WILTING THE CABBAGE IS THE KEY TO THIS SLAW. WE HAVE ALL HAD COLESLAW THAT LOOKS GREAT WHEN IT IS FIRST MADE, BUT SOON TURNS INTO A WATERY MESS. BY SALTING THE CABBAGE AHEAD OF TIME AND ALLOWING IT TO RELEASE WATER, YOU ENSURE THAT YOUR SLAW WILL HOLD ITS FORM AND FLAVOR.

1 head green cabbage, thinly shredded

$^1/_2$ teaspoon sea salt

1 cup (235 ml) apple cider vinegar

$^3/_4$ cup (180 ml) light olive oil

1 tablespoon (6.5 g) celery seed

2 tablespoons (18 g) dry mustard

1 red onion, thinly shaved

3 stalks celery, thinly sliced

2 medium carrots, grated

Mix the thinly sliced cabbage with the sea salt and transfer to a plastic container with a secure lid. Refrigerate overnight. The next day, remove from the refrigerator and strain the cabbage in a large colander. In a large mixing bowl, whisk together the vinegar, light olive oil, celery seed, and dry mustard. Add to this mixture the thinly shaved onion, celery, carrots, and cabbage. Mix thoroughly and refrigerate for 1 hour.

YIELD: 4 TO 8 SERVINGS

YAM, BACON, AND LIME IS A COMBINATION THAT ALLOWS YOU TO USE ALL OF YOUR PALATE. THE BACON BRINGS A SLIGHTLY SALTY ELEMENT, THE YAMS ARE SOMEWHAT SWEET, AND THE LIME IS A BIT SOUR.

1 pound (454 g) yams, peeled and diced

$^1/_2$ cup (125 g) Paleo Mayo (page 47)

4 ounces (112 g) bacon, cooked until crispy and drained

1 medium yellow onion, diced small

Juice of $^1/_2$ lime

2 tablespoons (8 g) chopped fresh tarragon

Freshly ground black pepper

1 $^1/_2$ teaspoons snipped fresh chives

Place the yams in a large pot and cover with cold water by at least 1 inch (2.5 cm). Bring to a simmer over medium heat, adjusting the temperature to never allow the water to come to a rolling boil. Once the water has come to a simmer, check the sweet potatoes for doneness by sticking with a fork every 15 to 20 minutes. They are done when the fork goes through easily without the yam completely falling apart or becoming mushy. Strain in a large colander and let cool at room temperature about 20 minutes. When there is no more steam but they are somewhat warm, transfer to a large mixing bowl.

Fold in the mayo, bacon, onion, lime juice, and tarragon. Season with black pepper and garnish with fresh chives. Let cool in the refrigerator for 2 to 4 hours.

YIELD: 4 TO 6 SERVINGS

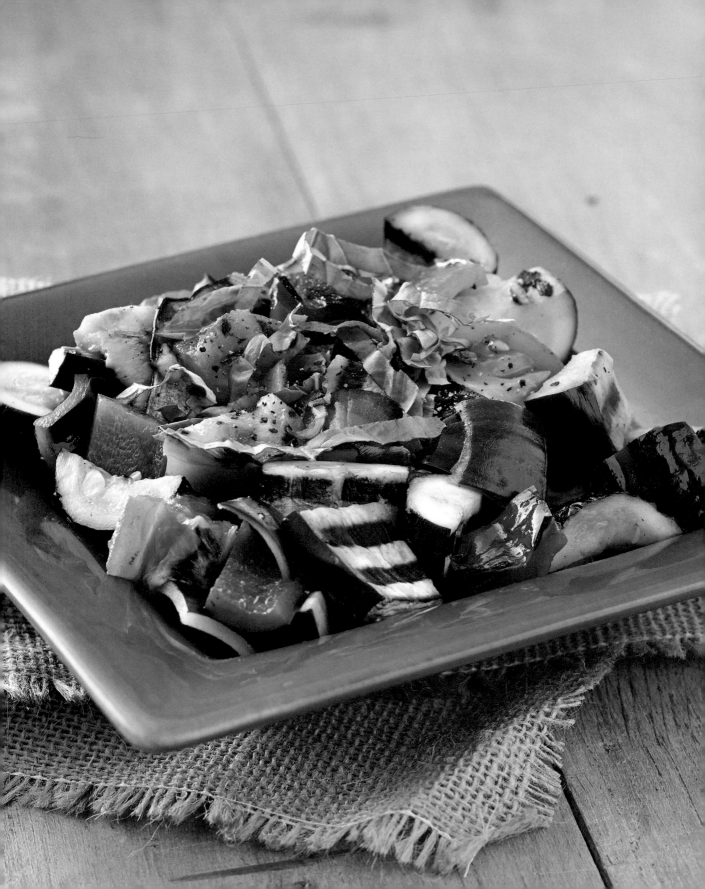

2 red onions, unpeeled

2 red bell peppers

2 green bell peppers

2 large tomatoes

4 cloves garlic, peeled and left whole

¼ cup (60 ml) extra virgin olive oil

1 large zucchini

1 large eggplant

¼ cup (60 ml) red wine vinegar

2 tablespoons (5 g) fresh basil, cut into fine ribbons

Salt and pepper to taste

ESCALIVADA

THIS ROASTED VEGETABLE DISH COMES FROM THE CATALONIA REGION OF SPAIN. ITS NAME COMES FROM THE WORD *ESCALIVAR,* WHICH MEANS "TO ROAST OVER ASHES OR EMBERS." IT IS A TRADITIONAL ACCOMPANIMENT, BUT ITS RICH TEXTURE AND SMOKY FLAVOR MAKE IT PERFECT AS A STAND-ALONE DISH AS WELL.

Preheat the grill to medium-high heat. Wash all the vegetables thoroughly. Place the whole, unpeeled red onions on the outside of the grate over indirect heat. Allow to cook until the outside is slightly charred and the onions are somewhat soft, about 1 hour. When the onions are finished, remove from the heat and allow to cool. When cooled, remove and discard the outer charred layers.

While the onions are cooking, place the whole peppers and tomatoes directly over the flames, rotating frequently with tongs. Remove when the skins of the peppers and tomatoes are slightly charred. Set aside and allow to cool, then peel the skin under running water. Cut the peppers and tomatoes in half and remove the seeds, cores, and stems. Place the garlic and olive oil in a small saucepan and cook over medium-low heat until the garlic is golden brown and fork-tender. Set aside and allow to cool.

Remove the ends of the whole zucchini and eggplant and cut lengthwise into ¼-inch (6 mm)-thick planks, rub with olive oil, season with salt and pepper, and grill until cooked through. Remove from the heat and allow to cool. When all of the vegetables have cooled, cut into uniform strips. Combine the vegetables in a mixing bowl and add the remaining garlic oil (with garlic), red wine vinegar, and basil. Season with salt and pepper to taste. Mix thoroughly.

YIELD: 6 TO 8 SERVINGS

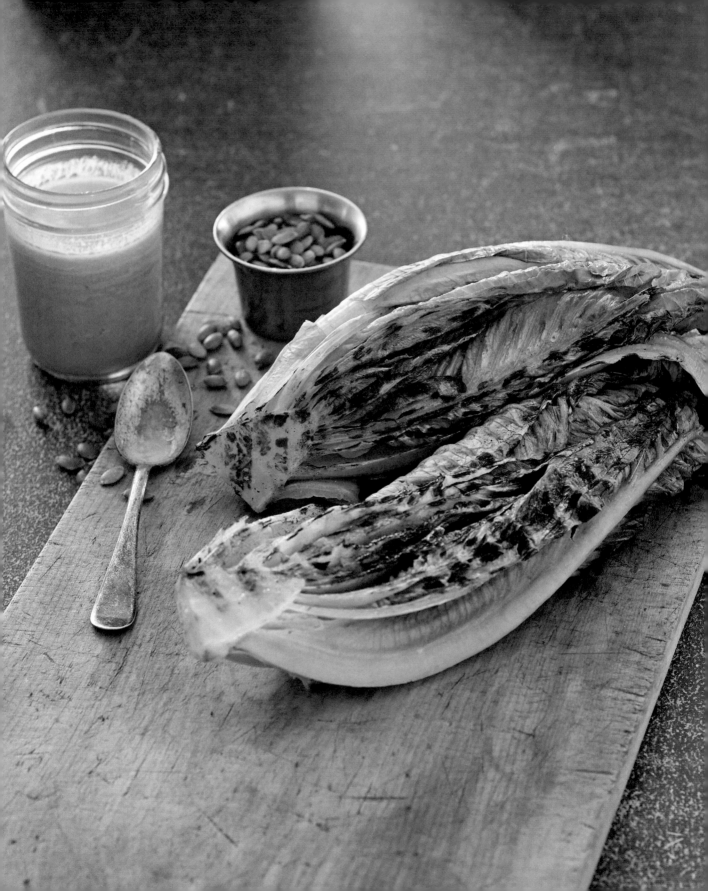

BLACKENED CAESAR SALAD

FOR CAESAR DRESSING:

1 can (2 ounces, or 54 g) anchovy fillets packed in olive oil, drained

1 clove garlic

Sea salt

2 large egg yolks

2 tablespoons (30 ml) fresh lemon juice

$^3/_4$ teaspoon Dijon mustard

2 tablespoons (30 ml) extra virgin olive oil

$^1/_2$ cup (120 ml) light olive oil

Freshly ground black pepper

FOR SALAD:

2 large heads romaine lettuce, cut lengthwise

Extra virgin olive oil

4 tablespoons (28 g) roasted pumpkin seeds

TO MAKE THE DRESSING: Add the anchovy fillets, garlic, and a pinch of sea salt to a food processor and pulse until combined. Turn the food processor on low and add the egg yolks, lemon juice, and Dijon mustard. Add the extra virgin olive oil in a slow drizzle until combined. Add the light olive oil, processing until thick and well combined. If desired, season with additional sea salt, freshly ground black pepper, and more lemon juice. Store in the refrigerator.

TO MAKE THE SALAD: Preheat your grill to medium-high and brush the cut surface of the romaine lettuce with olive oil. When the grill is hot, place the lettuce over direct heat, turning occasionally, for 4 to 5 minutes. When done, the lettuce will be slightly charred and tender. Place each lettuce half on a plate, drizzle with the Caesar dressing, and garnish with the roasted pumpkin seeds.

YIELD: 4 SERVINGS

GRILLED FENNEL AND RED ONION SALAD

2 red onions, unpeeled

2 bulbs fennel, stems removed, fronds reserved

1 English cucumber, peeled and thinly sliced at an angle

2 ripe avocados, peeled, pitted, and sliced $^1/_8$ inch (3 mm) lengthwise

1 tablespoon (4 g) fresh tarragon

$^1/_4$ cup (60 ml) White Balsamic Vinaigrette (page 52)

THIS IS A VEGETABLE-LOVER'S SALAD. IT IS HEARTY, REFRESHING, AND PERFECT FOR A HOT SUMMER AFTERNOON AROUND THE GRILL.

Preheat the grill to medium-high heat. Place the red onions on the hottest part of the grill and grill for 10 minutes. Roll the onions over and grill for another 10 minutes. When done, the outside should be charred and they should start to soften. Move the onions to the rack above the grill and place the fennel bulbs over the flame. Grill the fennel for 2 minutes on each side. Remove the fennel and onions from the heat. Place them on a platter and refrigerate until completely cool.

Peel the charred outside of the red onions and cut off the ends. Cut the onions and fennel in half and then slice into strips. Combine all of the ingredients in a mixing bowl and toss. Arrange in a serving bowl.

YIELD: 4 OR 5 SERVINGS

GRILLED VEGETABLE GAZPACHO ANDALUZ

2 beefsteak tomatoes

1 red bell pepper

1 yellow bell pepper

$^1/_2$ medium red onion, peeled and cut into $^1/_4$-inch (6 mm) rings

1 English cucumber, peeled and chopped

1 clove garlic

1 small bunch cilantro, washed, dried, and rough chopped

$^1/_4$ cup (60 ml) extra virgin olive oil

2 tablespoons (30 ml) sherry vinegar

1 teaspoon black pepper

Pinch of sea salt

$^1/_4$ cup (65 g) Ajo Blanco (page 47)

1 ounce (28 g) almond slivers, toasted

THIS COOL AND RICHLY FLAVORED SOUP OWES ITS ROOTS TO SPANISH CUISINE AND HOT SUMMER NIGHTS.

Preheat the grill to high. Core the tomatoes and cut them in half. Place them on the grill, flesh side down. Place the peppers and onion rings over the flame. Grill the onions and tomatoes for 3 minutes on each side and remove from the grill. The peppers will take about 10 minutes longer. Rotate and turn the peppers every few minutes until the skin is completely charred. Remove them from the grill and place in a mixing bowl. Cover the bowl tightly with plastic wrap and set aside for 10 minutes.

Using a clean, dry towel, wipe away the black skin from the outside of the peppers. Break open the peppers and discard the stem and seeds. Roughly chop the grilled vegetables and add to a blender. Be sure to scrape all of the juices from the cutting board into the blender as well. Add the cucumber, garlic, cilantro, oil, vinegar, pepper, and salt and blend, pulsing at first, then on high for 3 to 4 minutes. Pour into a shallow container and cool for 2 to 5 hours.

Divide among 4 bowls, garnish with the ajo blanco and toasted almond slivers, and serve.

YIELD: 4 SERVINGS

SMOKY MUSHROOM AND HERB SOUP

FOR SOUP STOCK:

1 pound (454 g) oak wood chunks, soaked in water for 1 hour

2 chicken carcasses

2 yellow onions, cut in half

1 head celery

2 carrots, cut in half

2 heads garlic

1 whole fennel bulb

1 gallon (3.8 L) cold water

4 ounces (112 g) fresh thyme

1¹/₂ teaspoons whole peppercorns

FOR SOUP:

2 large portobello mushrooms caps (stems reserved for stock)

10 to 15 shiitake mushroom caps (stems reserved for stock)

1 bunch parsley, rinsed, dried, and finely chopped (stems reserved for stock)

1 ounce (28 g) basil (stems removed and sliced into thin strips and reserved for stock)

2 tablespoons (30 ml) extra virgin olive oil

GRILLED MUSHROOMS AND SMOKED VEGETABLES ADD FIRE TO THIS CLASSIC COMBINATION OF FLAVORS. USING THE WHOLE CHICKEN CARCASS ALSO ENSURES THAT THE SOUP STOCK WILL HAVE A VELVETY TEXTURE.

TO MAKE THE SOUP STOCK: Preheat the coals in the grill to high heat with the oak spread evenly over them. When the oak starts to smoke, place the chicken carcasses, onions, celery, carrots, garlic, and fennel bulb on the grill and close the lid. Smoke for 10 minutes. Transfer the bones and vegetables to a large stockpot and place the pot on the stove. Pour the cold water over the bones and vegetables and turn the heat on high.

When the stock comes to a simmer, use a large spoon to skim off the foam that forms on top. Turn the heat to low and add the thyme, peppercorns, reserved mushroom stems, and reserved herb stems. The stock should simmer but not boil. Check it periodically and skim when necessary. Cook for 1 hour.

Drizzle the mushroom caps with the light olive oil and season with black pepper. Place the mushroom caps on the grill and cover for 5 minutes. Remove the lid and turn the mushrooms over. Grill with the lid closed for another 5 minutes. Remove the mushrooms from the grill and when they are cool enough to handle, cut into medium-size chunks.

When the stock is finished, strain it through a fine sieve and into a double boiler to keep warm. If you don't have a double boiler, simply put a smaller stockpot into a larger pot. Fill the larger pot with enough water to come about halfway up the sides of the smaller pot and put both pots on a burner set to medium-low heat.

TO MAKE THE SOUP: Put a portion of smoked mushrooms into each serving bowl and sprinkle the fresh parsley and basil leaves over the mushrooms. Ladle hot stock over the mushrooms and herbs and drizzle with the extra virgin olive oil.

YIELD: 6 TO 8 SERVINGS

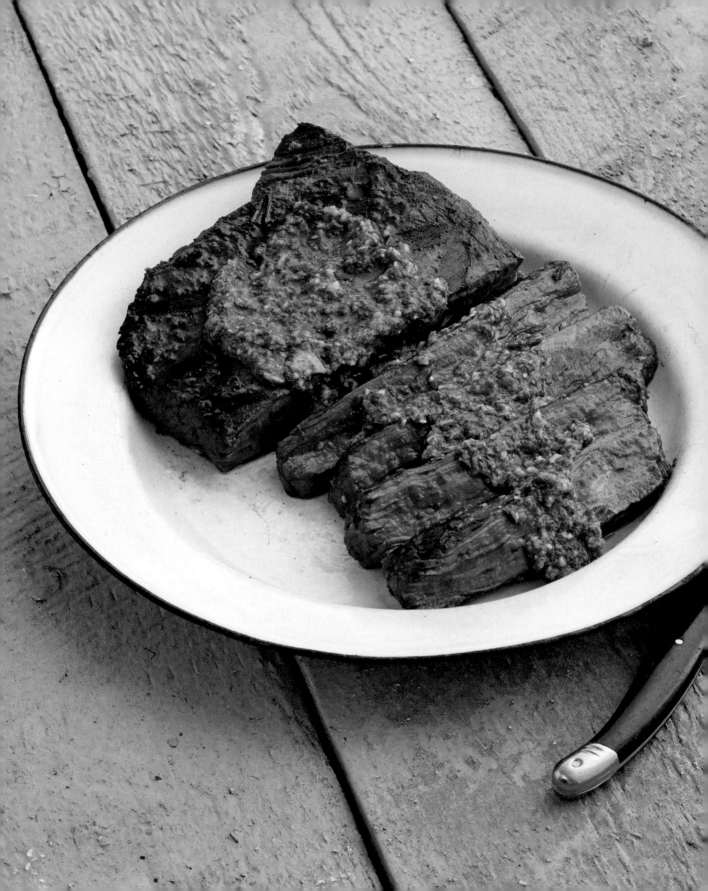

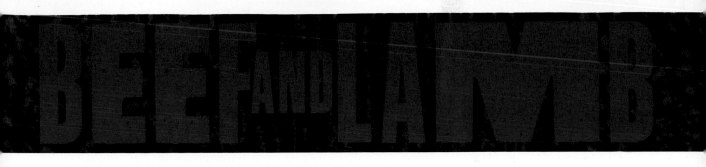

½ cup (120 ml) coconut aminos

½ cup (120 ml) extra virgin olive oil

Juice of 2 limes

2 teaspoons (5 g) smoked paprika

6 large cloves garlic, minced

2 tablespoons (3 g) chopped fresh rosemary

2 tablespoons (5 g) chopped fresh thyme

2 tablespoons (12 g) coarsely ground black pepper

1 teaspoon sea salt

2 to 2½ pounds (0.9 to 1.1 kg) flank steak

1 cup (240 g) Escalivada (page 67), for garnish

4 tablespoons (60 g) Chimichurri (page 51), for topping

GRILLED FLANK STEAK
WITH ESCALIVADA AND CHIMICHURRI

FLANK STEAK COMES FROM THE ABDOMINAL MUSCLES OF THE COW AND IS A COMMON CUT OF BEEF IN COLOMBIA, WHERE IT IS KNOWN AS *SOBREBARRIGA,* WHICH TRANSLATES TO "OVER THE BELLY." IT CAN BE TOUGH IF HANDLED IMPROPERLY, BUT WITH PROPER PREPARATION, IT CAN BE COAXED INTO TENDERNESS. IN THIS RECIPE, FLANK STEAK IS MARINATED WITH HERBS AND SPICES TO DRIVE FLAVOR DEEP INTO THE MEAT. WHEN SERVED, ITS RICH BEEFINESS IS COMPLEMENTED BY SPICY CHIMICHURRI AND ROASTED VEGETABLE ESCALIVADA.

Combine the coconut aminos, oil, lime juice, paprika, garlic, rosemary, thyme, pepper, and salt in a 13 x 9-inch (33 x 23 cm) glass baking dish. Add the steak and turn to coat. Cover and refrigerate for 2 hours, turning occasionally.

Preheat the grill to high. Remove the meat from the marinade and grill to desired doneness, about 4 minutes per side for medium-rare. Flank steak shouldn't be cooked over medium-rare or it will be tough. Transfer the steak to a cutting board and let rest for 5 minutes. Cut across the grain into thin strips.

Arrange the escalivada on a platter and lay the flank strips over the top. Top with a generous amount of chimichurri and serve.

YIELD: 4 TO 6 SERVINGS

¹/₄ cup (60 g) olive oil

4 cloves garlic, minced

1 tablespoon (1.7 g) chopped
fresh rosemary

1 tablespoon (1 g) chopped
fresh cilantro

1 teaspoon sweet paprika

1 teaspoon red pepper flakes

Juice of 2 limes

Salt and freshly
ground black pepper

2¹/₂-pound (1.1 kg) tri-tip steak

4 tablespoons (65 g) Charred
Tomatillo Salsa (page 47),
for topping

FOR DECADES, THE TERM *TRI-TIP* WAS RARELY USED OUTSIDE OF CALIFORNIA, THE FIRST AREA WHERE THIS TRIANGULAR CUT OF THE ROAST FIRST BECAME POPULAR. (IT'S REFERRED TO AS THE "TRI-TIP" BECAUSE THE ROAST COMES FROM THE INTERSECTION OF THE SIRLOIN, FLANK, AND ROUND PRIMALS.) RECENTLY, THIS CUT, KNOWN FOR ITS FLAVOR AND MARBLING, HAS BECOME POPULAR ACROSS THE COUNTRY. IT'S PRACTICALLY MADE FOR THE GRILL.

Place the oil, garlic, rosemary, cilantro, paprika, red pepper flakes, and lime juice in a small bowl and stir to combine. Allow the flavors to infuse for 2 hours. Rub a generous amount of salt and pepper all over the tri-tip, followed by the marinade. Marinate the tri-tip for 2 to 4 hours. Transfer the tri-tip to a baking sheet and let sit at room temperature while you prepare the grill.

Preheat the grill to high. Place the tri-tip on the grill over the coals, cover the grill, and cook for 3 minutes. Rotate the tri-tip 90 degrees (keeping the meat over the coals), cover, and grill until the underside is deep brown and grill marks have appeared, about 2 to 3 minutes more. Flip the tri-tip and continue grilling over the coals, rotating 90 degrees once during the cooking time, until the meat is deep brown, grill marks have appeared, and the tri-tip has reached an internal temperature of 125°F (51°C) for medium-rare, about 9 to 12 minutes total. Transfer the meat to a cutting board, and let rest for 8 to 10 minutes. Slice against the grain and top with salsa.

YIELD: 4 TO 6 SERVINGS

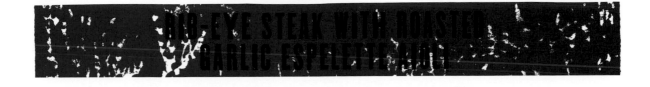

FOR ROASTED GARLIC ESPELETTE AIOLI:

1 large head garlic

1 tablespoon (15 ml) olive oil

Salt and pepper

2 cups (520 g) Paleo Mayo (page 47)

$^1/_2$ teaspoon espelette or other ground chile pepper

FOR STEAK:

4 steaks (10 to 12 ounces, or 280 to 336 g, each) prime or choice beef rib-eye, 1 inch (2.5 cm) thick

1 tablespoon (15 ml) olive oil

Coarsely ground sea salt

Freshly ground black pepper

1 tablespoon (4.3 g) dried thyme

ESPELETTE IS A GROUND RED CHILE PEPPER THAT IS USED IN FRANCE IN PLACE OF BLACK PEPPER. IN THIS RECIPE, IT GIVES THE AIOLI TOPPING A FIERY KICK TO COMPLEMENT THE RICH FLAVOR OF THE RIB EYE.

TO MAKE THE AIOLI: Preheat the oven to 300°F (150°C, or gas mark 2). Cut a thin slice off the very top of the head of garlic to expose the tops of all the cloves. Set the garlic head in a shallow baking dish. Pour the oil slowly over and into the head. Season with the salt and pepper. Cover the pan with aluminum foil and bake for 1 hour, until the garlic is somewhat soft and golden brown. Drain and reserve the oil. Set the garlic aside.

When cool, squeeze the pulp out of the roasted garlic and fold into the mayo. Add the espelette and stir to combine.

TO MAKE THE STEAK: Preheat the grill to medium-high heat. Rub the rib eye with the olive oil and generously season with the salt and pepper. Sprinkle with the thyme and place on the grill. Allow to sear for 4 to 6 minutes, turn 90 degrees, and sear for another 4 to 6 minutes. Flip the steaks and repeat on the other side. When the steak has an internal temperature of 125°F (51°C), remove from the grill and allow to rest for 10 minutes. Top with the aioli and serve.

YIELD: 4 SERVINGS

"My favorite animal is steak." **—FRAN LEBOWITZ**

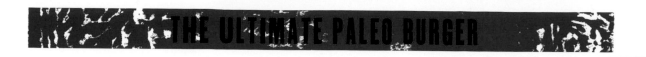

FOR BURGERS:

¹/₂ pound (226 g) ground sirloin

¹/₂ pound (226 g) ground chuck

1 teaspoon Worcestershire sauce

1 teaspoon minced garlic

¹/₂ medium white onion, minced

Freshly ground black pepper

Sea salt

FOR TOPPINGS AND BURGER "BUN":

8 slices bacon

¹/₂ medium white onion, thinly sliced

2 eggs

1 head iceberg lettuce

2 tablespoons (32 g) Paleo Mayo (page 47)

1 tablespoon (15 g) Kicked-Up Ketchup (page 46)

1 tablespoon (11 g) yellow mustard

¹/₂ cup (118 g) bread and butter pickles

BITE OFF A PIECE OF AWESOME PACKED WITH KILLER TOPPINGS. THE GROUND CHUCK AND SIRLOIN WILL KEEP THIS BURGER MOIST THANKS TO THE FAT IN THE CHUCK AND FLAVORFUL DUE TO THE RICH SIRLOIN. WRAPPING THIS BABY IN LETTUCE KICKS WHEAT BUNS TO THE CURB.

TO MAKE THE BURGERS: In a large bowl, combine the ground sirloin, ground chuck, Worcestershire sauce, garlic, and minced onion. Crack in a generous amount of fresh black pepper and season with a good pinch of sea salt. Combine the mixture well and form into 2 patties.

TO PREPARE THE TOPPINGS AND "BUN": Get your grill nice and hot and, using a cast-iron skillet, fry up the strips of bacon until crispy. Remove the bacon and use the bacon fat to fry the sliced onion. The onions should take about 20 minutes to get really caramelized.

Cook the burgers on direct high heat. Whatever you do, don't press on them with your spatula. Pressing on burgers only squeezes out the juice, which is a stupid thing to do if you want a juicy burger. Flip the burgers after 4 or 5 minutes and cook for an additional 4 or 5 minutes or less if you want them on the rare side.

When the burgers are done cooking, put them on a plate to rest. Remove the caramelized onions from the skillet and use the remaining fat in the pan to fry up the eggs.

Prepare the "buns" by cutting the head of lettuce in half, removing several layers of the largest leaves. Place a piece of parchment paper down and put a stack of iceberg lettuce leaves on top of it. Put down the burger patty and dress with the Paleo Mayo, Kicked-Up Ketchup, and mustard. Add the pickles and bacon on top of the condiments, saving the fried egg for the very top. Cap the burger with another stack of iceberg lettuce leaves. Use the parchment paper to wrap the burger up, folding the paper first from the bottom and then from the sides. Repeat this process for the second burger and high-five your dining partner.

YIELD: 2 SERVINGS

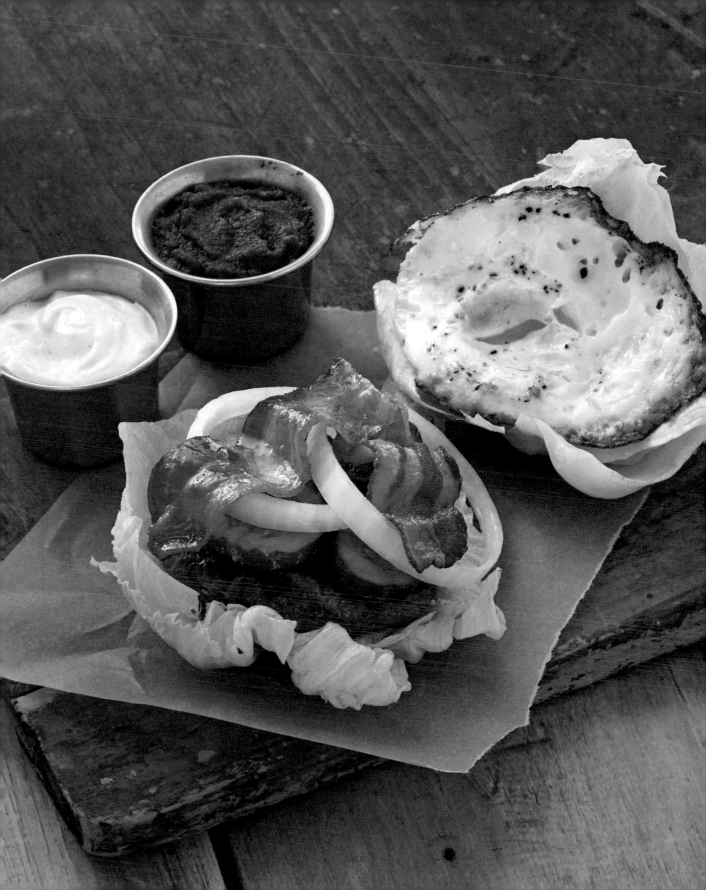

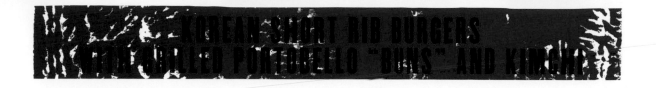

FOR PORTOBELLO "BUNS":

6 large portobello mushrooms, stems removed

Olive oil

Sea salt and black pepper

FOR BURGERS:

1¹/₂ pounds (680 g) ground short rib meat or 80/20 ground meat

1 tablespoon (10 g) finely minced garlic

1 teaspoon red pepper flakes

1 teaspoon minced pickled ginger

2 scallions, thinly sliced

2 tablespoons (30 ml) rice wine (dry sherry can be substituted if rice wine is unavailable)

1¹/₂ teaspoons toasted sesame oil

¹/₂ teaspoon coarsely ground sea salt

¹/₂ teaspoon freshly ground black pepper

THE KOREAN DISH KNOWN AS *GALBI* IS TRADITIONALLY PREPARED WITH THINLY SLICED, MARINATED PIECES OF SHORT RIB. BY FUSING THE FLAVORS OF THIS DISH INTO A BURGER, TOPPING IT WITH KIMCHI, AND WRAPPING IT IN PORTOBELLO MUSHROOM "BUNS," YOU'LL GET SOMETHING THAT'S ONE PART FAMILIAR, ONE PART DIFFERENT, AND TWO PARTS DELICIOUS. ALSO, THE PROBIOTICS IN RAW KIMCHI ARE BENEFICIAL FOR THE DIGESTIVE SYSTEM AND MAY EVEN HELP WITH AUTOIMMUNE DISORDERS. KIMCHI IS AVAILABLE AT ASIAN GROCERS AS WELL AS MANY SUPERMARKETS.

TO MAKE THE BUNS: Preheat the grill to medium-high heat and arrange the coals so that one side of the grill will provide direct heat and the other indirect. Drizzle the mushroom caps with the olive oil and season with salt and pepper. Arrange the mushrooms cap side down on the half of the grill providing indirect heat. Close the lid of the grill and allow the mushrooms to cook for 15 to 20 minutes. When the mushrooms are tender, transfer to a paper towel–lined plate and cover until ready to serve.

TO MAKE THE BURGERS: Combine the ground short rib meat in a large bowl with all of the other ingredients. Form into 3 large burgers and place on the side of the grill providing direct heat. Cook the burgers to medium-rare (internal temperature of 125°F [51°C]) before removing them to a plate to rest.

"Sacred cows make the best hamburger." **—MARK TWAIN**

FOR TOPPING:

1 cup (140 g) kimchi

1 ounce (28 g) thinly sliced red onion

1 ounce (28 g) shredded carrot

2 ounces (56 g) fresh napa cabbage, thinly shredded

TO PREPARE THE TOPPINGS: Take one of the portobello mushroom buns and turn it gill side up. Place a burger on top of the mushroom and top with a portion of the kimchi. Add a few slices of red onion, some carrot, and a portion of fresh napa cabbage. Top the burger with another portobello mushroom bun and wrap halfway with butcher paper or foil.

YIELD: 3 SERVINGS

CAN I MAKE KIMCHI AT HOME?

Kimchi is easy to make and nearly foolproof. You simply need a sealable glass or ceramic container, cabbage, scallion, garlic, ginger, fish sauce, and red pepper flakes. Salt the cabbage to draw out the water, then mix with the other ingredients. Seal and leave on the counter for a day or two and there you have it! For more detailed instructions as well as information about the health benefits of kimchi, go to PerfectHealthDiet.com and search for "Homemade Kimchi."

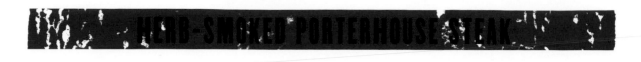

**FOR BEEF
TALLOW "BUTTER":**

3 cloves garlic, minced

¹/₄ teaspoon sea salt

2 cups (410 g) beef tallow

**¹/₂ teaspoon Worcestershire
sauce**

¹/₄ teaspoon black pepper

**1 tablespoon (2.4 g) chopped
fresh thyme**

FOR STEAK:

1 bunch fresh thyme

1 bunch fresh sage

3 sprigs fresh rosemary

**3- to 4-pound (1.4 to 1.8 kg)
porterhouse steak**

1 tablespoon (15 ml) olive oil

**1 tablespoon (18 g) coarsely
ground sea salt**

1 tablespoon (18 g) smoked salt

**1 tablespoon (6 g) coarsely
ground black pepper**

HERB SMOKING IS NOT SOMETHING YOU SEE DONE VERY OFTEN, BUT IT IMPARTS AN INCREDIBLE AND UNIQUE FLAVOR. THE INTENSITY OF THE SMOKE CAN BE FAIRLY POWERFUL, WHICH WORKS WITH BIG CUTS SUCH AS A PORTERHOUSE.

TO PREPARE THE BEEF TALLOW "BUTTER": Make a paste out of the garlic and sea salt (use either a mortar and pestle or the flat blade of a chef's knife against a cutting board). Soften the beef tallow in a bath of warm water (make sure none of the water gets into the tallow itself). Thoroughly combine the garlic paste, tallow, Worcestershire, pepper, and thyme. Place on a large piece of parchment paper and form it into a log shape. Roll the mixture with the parchment paper and twist the ends to seal. Place in the refrigerator until firm.

TO MAKE THE STEAK: Prepare the herbs for smoking by first soaking them in cool water for 10 minutes. Preheat the grill to low. Lift up the grill grate and put half of the soaked herbs into your gas grill's smoker box or directly onto coals if using charcoal. They should immediately start to smoke.

Rub the steak with the olive oil and sprinkle with the salts and pepper. Place the steak on the grill and close the lid. After approximately 8 minutes, open the grill and rotate the steak 90 degrees. Close the lid and cook for another 8 minutes. Open the lid and put the remaining soaked herbs onto the coals or into the smoker box. Flip the steak and cook for 8 more minutes, then rotate 90 degrees, and cook for a final 8 minutes. Check the internal temperature of the steak with an instant-read thermometer; it should be about 125°F (51°C) for medium-rare.

Top the steak with a generous medallion of beef tallow "butter" and let the steak rest for 5 minutes before slicing across the grain and serving.

YIELD: 4 TO 6 SERVINGS

FOR CAPER HAZELNUT PERSILLADE:

¹/₄ cup (30 g) hazelnuts

¹/₂ cup (30 g) minced fresh flat-leaf parsley

¹/₄ cup (12 g) minced chives

2 teaspoons (2.5 g) minced tarragon

1 teaspoon minced chervil

2 oil-packed anchovy fillets, minced

2 teaspoons (6 g) capers, rinsed and chopped

1 medium shallot, minced

2 tablespoons (30 ml) sherry vinegar

³/₄ cup (175 ml) extra virgin olive oil, plus more for brushing

Salt and freshly ground pepper

FOR STEAK:

2 trimmed 1-pound (454 g) hanger steaks

2 tablespoons (30 ml) olive oil

1 tablespoon (18 g) sea salt

1 tablespoon (6 g) cracked black pepper

HANGER STEAK IS A LOW-COST, FLAVORFUL CUT THAT IS BEST WHEN COOKED RARE OR MEDIUM-RARE. ANYTHING OVER MEDIUM-RARE CAN CAUSE THE MEAT TO BE TOUGH AND SOMEWHAT STRINGY.

TO MAKE THE PERSILLADE: Preheat the oven to 375ºF (190ºC, or gas mark 5). Toast the hazelnuts in a pie plate for 12 minutes, or until the skins are blistered. Transfer the nuts to a kitchen towel; let cool slightly, then rub off the skins. Finely chop the nuts and transfer them to a bowl. Add the parsley, chives, tarragon, chervil, anchovies, capers, and shallot. Stir in the vinegar and oil and season with salt and pepper.

TO MAKE THE STEAK: Preheat the grill to medium-high heat or preheat a grill pan. Brush the steaks with the oil and season generously with the salt and pepper. Grill, turning occasionally, for about 12 minutes for medium-rare. Let the meat rest for 5 minutes. Slice the meat across the grain and serve with the persillade.

YIELD: 4 SERVINGS

2 tablespoons (10 g) mixed whole peppercorns

2 steaks (1 pound, or 454 g, each) well-marbled prime New York strip

2 tablespoons (28 g) beef tallow

Sea salt

THIS IS A PALEO TAKE ON THE CLASSIC DISH STEAK AU POIVRE, A PEPPER-CRUSTED STEAK THAT IS A STAPLE OF FRENCH CUISINE.

Coarsely grind the peppercorns in a mortar and pestle or spice grinder. Place the ground peppercorns on a plate. Rub the steaks with the tallow and then press firmly into the ground peppercorns, ensuring that the steaks are coated evenly on both sides. Season generously with sea salt.

Use additional tallow to lubricate the grill grate and then heat your grill to medium-high heat. Add the steaks to the grill and allow to cook over direct heat for about 1^1/$_2$ minutes, then turn the steaks 90 degrees and cook for an additional 1 minute. Flip the steaks and repeat on the other side. When done, the internal temperature should be about 130°F (54°C) for medium-rare, 135°F (57°C) for medium, 145°F (63°C) for medium-well, and 150°F (66°C) for well.

YIELD: 4 SERVINGS

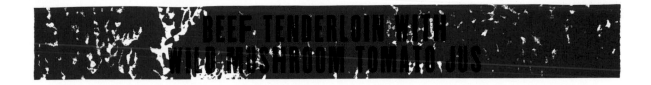

BEEF TENDERLOIN WITH WILD MUSHROOM TOMATO JUS

FOR WILD MUSHROOM TOMATO JUS:

1 quart (940 ml) veal or beef stock

8 dry-packed sun-dried tomatoes, thinly sliced

1 teaspoon avocado oil

15 chanterelle or shiitake mushrooms, thinly sliced

2 shallots, thinly sliced

1 tablespoon (4 g) coarsely chopped fresh Italian parsley, divided

1 teaspoon fresh thyme, divided

4 cloves garlic, roasted

FOR TENDELOIN:

4 medallions (5 to 6 ounces, or 140 to 170 g, each) beef tenderloin

Avocado oil

Sea salt and black pepper

THIS IS A CLASSIC DISH FOR THOSE TIMES WHEN YOU WANT TO BE IMMERSED IN FLAVOR. IT IS EARTHY, RICH, SWEET, AND BRIGHT. YOUR PALATE WILL BE STIMULATED WITH EVERY BITE.

TO MAKE THE JUS: Add the stock to a large pan and bring to a boil over high heat. Reduce the heat to a simmer and allow to reduce for 35 to 40 minutes (or until three-fourths of the original amount remains). Turn off the heat and add the tomatoes. Allow to steep for 30 minutes.

In another pot, heat the avocado oil until almost smoking (the oil is ready when a drop of water sputters and steams immediately after being dropped into the pan). Add the mushrooms and shallots. Sauté while stirring for 2 minutes, or until golden brown. Remove from the heat.

Add the stock to the mushrooms and shallots while tilting the pot away from you. The stock will splatter if added too quickly or over too high a heat. Allow to return to a simmer and turn off the heat. Add half of the parsley and thyme and the roasted garlic.

TO MAKE THE TENDERLOIN: Preheat the grill to medium-high heat. Brush the beef lightly with the avocado oil, then sprinkle with the salt, pepper, and the remaining half of the herbs. Place the beef medallions on the grill and cook without moving for 2 minutes. Turn the medallions 90 degrees and cook for another 2 minutes. Flip the medallions and repeat on the other side. When done, the internal temperature should be 130°F (54°C) for medium-rare, 135°F (57°C) for medium, 145°F (63°C) for medium-well, and 150°F (66°C) for well. Allow the medallions to rest for 5 minutes.

Spoon the jus over the top of each medallion and serve.

YIELD: 4 SERVINGS

A WORD ABOUT MUSHROOMS

Special care should be taken to properly prepare mushrooms. Chanterelles should be cleaned and dried thoroughly and trimmed at the stem end and shiitakes should be destemmed before using.

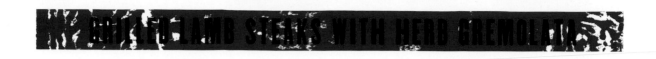
GRILLED LAMB STEAKS WITH HERB GREMOLATA

**2 lamb sirloin steaks
(2¹/₂ pounds, or 1.1 kg each)**

**2 cups (200 g) Gremolata
(page 51)**

WHEN MOST PEOPLE THINK OF STEAKS, THEY AUTOMATICALLY THINK OF BEEF, BUT LAMB STEAKS ARE GREAT ON THE GRILL AS WELL! LAMB NATURALLY HAS A WONDERFUL FLAVOR, BUT PAIRING IT WITH THIS FRESH HERB GREMOLATA REALLY MAKES THIS DISH. THIS RECIPE COMES COURTESY OF KEITH AND MICHELLE NORRIS, ORGANIZERS OF PALEOFX (PALEOFX.COM) AND OWNERS OF INSTINCT CATERING AND EVENTS.

Preheat your grill to high heat. Place the lamb steaks on the grill over direct heat. Let the steaks sear for about 3 minutes before rotating 90 degrees (to get those perfect grill marks). Cook for an additional 3 minutes before flipping the steaks and repeating the process. When done, the outside should be very slightly charred, but the inside should be rare to medium-rare. Transfer the steaks to a cutting board and allow to rest for 5 minutes before carving. Serve the carved steak topped with the Gremolata.

YIELD: 6 TO 8 SERVINGS

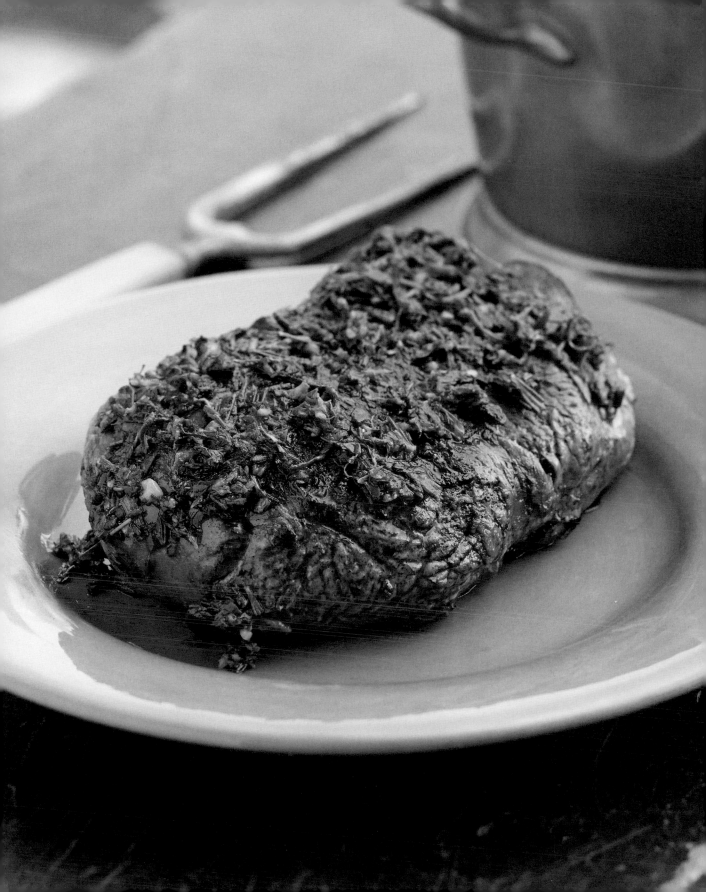

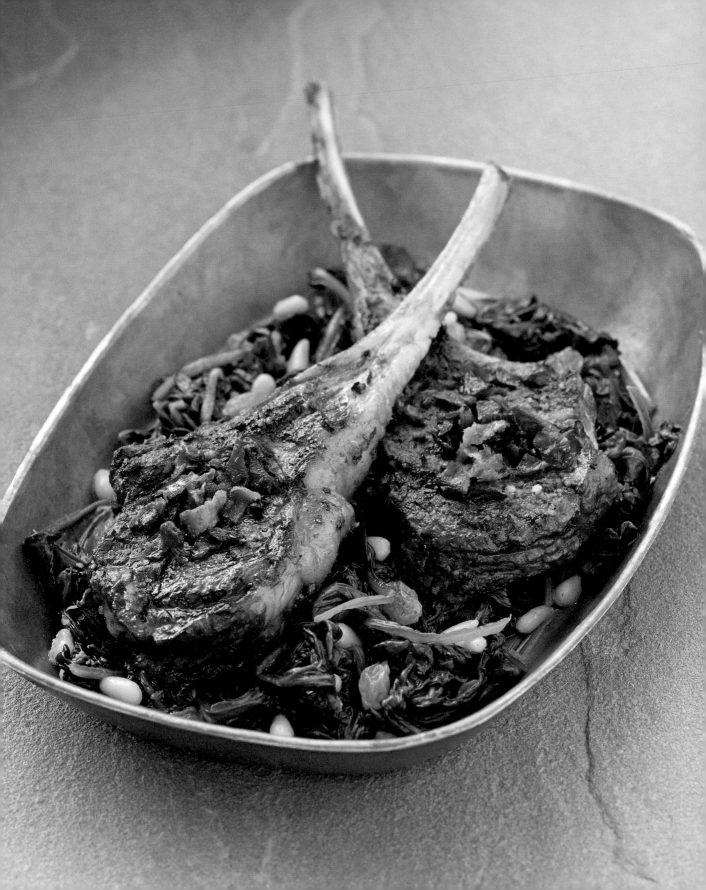

8 cloves garlic, roasted

2 anchovy fillets

1 teaspoon smoked paprika

Zest of 1 lemon

4 tablespoons (15 g) chopped
Italian parsley

6 tablespoons (90 ml) plus 1
teaspoon Spanish olive oil

One 8-bone rack of
lamb, trimmed

2 ounces (55 g) jamon serrano
(also sold as serrano ham)

1 shallot, minced

4 tablespoons (60 ml)
amontillado sherry

8 ounces (225 g) baby spinach

2 ounces (56 g) golden raisins

2 ounces (56 g)
pine nuts, toasted

Salt and black pepper

THE RACK OF LAMB IS A CULINARY CLASSIC THAT WILL WOW
YOUR GUESTS, ESPECIALLY WHEN PAIRED WITH A ZESTY, SAVORY,
SWEET, AND SALTY SERRANO HAM DRESSING.

In a mortar and pestle, combine the garlic, anchovies, paprika, lemon zest,
and parsley. Grind into a rough paste while gradually emulsifying with the
6 tablespoons (90 ml) olive oil. When fully incorporated, rub completely
over the trimmed rack of lamb. Wrap each bone with aluminum foil to
prevent charring. Marinate for 30 minutes at room temperature.

Make sure the grill is clean and lightly oiled. Preheat the grill to low
heat. Place the rack fatty side down on the grill. Be sure not to place it
directly over the flame because the high fat content of the cap will cause
it to flare. Remove from the heat as soon as flares occur. Slowly cook the
lamb at 250°F (120°C) for 12 to 15 minutes, turning once and flipping
over for another 3 to 5 minutes. The internal temperature of the rack
should be no higher than 125°F (51°C). Remove from the heat and allow
to rest for 10 minutes. Carve along the bones.

Heat the remaining 1 teaspoon olive oil in a sauté pan. Add the jamon
serrano and stir continuously until lightly browned and crispy, about 8
minutes. Remove from the pan with a slotted spoon and transfer to a
paper towel–lined plate.

Add the shallots to the pan and cook over medium-high heat, until
lightly sweating. When the shallots are translucent, deglaze with the
sherry and reduce by half. Add the spinach and wilt for 1 minute. Finish
with the raisins, pine nuts, salt, and pepper. Serve as a side for the grilled
lamb. Garnish with the crispy jamon serrano.

YIELD: 2 TO 4 SERVINGS

THE AROMATICS OF TARRAGON COMPLEMENT THE RICHNESS OF LAMB, AND POMEGRANATE ADDS SWEETNESS TO THE SALTY, SAVORY MEAT.

FROM ABEL JAMES, AKA "THE FAT-BURNING MAN," COMES THIS ANTIOXIDANT-, PROTEIN-, AND FLAVOR-RICH RECIPE FOR CURRIED LAMB BLADE CHOPS. CHECK OUT MORE OF ABEL'S FOOD, AND FOOD FOR THOUGHT, AT FATBURNINGMAN.COM.

FOR POMEGRANATE TARRAGON SAUCE:

¹/₂ cup (120 ml) pomegranate molasses (you can substitute coconut nectar if unavailable)

¹/₄ cup (60 ml) pomegranate juice

1 cinnamon stick

1 tablespoon (4 g) coarsely chopped fresh tarragon

FOR LAMB:

4- to 5-pound (1.8 to 2.3 kg) boneless leg of lamb, rolled and tied

Sea salt and black pepper

TO MAKE THE SAUCE: In a small saucepan, combine the pomegranate molasses, pomegranate juice, and cinnamon stick. Warm slowly over low heat for 20 minutes, or until the sauce has a thin, syrupy consistency. Stir in the tarragon. Use half of the sauce for basting and reserve half for serving.

TO MAKE THE LAMB: Preheat the grill to medium heat. While it heats up, unroll the lamb and brush on all sides with the pomegranate sauce, seasoning generously with salt and pepper. Retie the lamb with butcher's twine. Place the lamb over indirect heat and cook for 15 minutes. Baste with the sauce again and turn 90 degrees. Cook for another 15 minutes. Turn the lamb over and repeat on the other side. The lamb should cook for a total of 1 hour, or until it reaches an internal temperature of 125°F (51°C). Remove from the heat and allow to rest for 10 minutes. Using a sharp knife, cut the leg of lamb into ¹/₄-inch (6 mm) slices and serve with the reserved sauce.

YIELD: 12 TO 14 SERVINGS

1 teaspoon turmeric

1¹/₂ tablespoons (9 g) curry powder

1¹/₂ teaspoons (4.5 g) garlic powder

¹/₂ teaspoon cayenne pepper

1 teaspoon paprika

1 teaspoon onion flakes

1 teaspoon black pepper

1 teaspoon salt

2 lamb blade chops (8 to 10 ounces, or 228 to 280 g, each)

2 tablespoons (28 g) coconut oil

¹/₂ cup (120 ml) white wine

Mix all of the spices together in a bowl. Dip the lamb blade chops in the spice mixture to coat both sides. Reserve the remaining spices.

In a sauté pan, melt the coconut oil over medium heat. Add the reserved spices and cook for 1 minute while stirring. Deglaze the pan with the white wine and bring to a boil. Reduce the heat and cover.

Preheat the grill to high heat. Place the lamb on the grill and sear both sides, about 2 to 3 minutes per side, or until the desired doneness (145°F [63°C] for medium-rare, 160°F [71°C] for medium, and 170°F [77°C] for medium-well).

Drizzle the lamb chops with the sauce and serve.

YIELD: 2 SERVINGS

FOR RUB:

1 tablespoon (6 g) fennel seed, crushed

1 teaspoon juniper berries, crushed

1 teaspoon coriander seed, crushed

1 tablespoon (15 ml) extra virgin olive oil

4 tablespoons (8 g) chopped fresh rosemary

FOR LAMB:

2 loins (7 ounces, or 200 g each) boneless lamb, trimmed of fat and silver skin

Coarsely ground sea salt

Fresh ground black pepper

LOIN HAS A SMOOTH, UNIFORM TEXTURE THAT IS LEAN AND LENDS ITSELF TO RARE TEMPERATURES. LAMB LOIN SHOULD NOT BE COOKED PAST MEDIUM-RARE AND SHOULD BE WELL RESTED BEFORE SLICING. IT HAS A TENDENCY TO DRY OUT, SO PAY ATTENTION WHILE IT COOKS.

TO MAKE THE RUB: Using a spice grinder or mortar and pestle, coarsely grind the fennel, juniper, and coriander seeds. Combine with the oil and rosemary in a small mixing bowl.

TO MAKE THE LAMB: Rub the lamb loins with the spice rub, salt, and pepper and place in a glass dish. Wrap in plastic and put in the refrigerator, marinating for at least 3 hours or overnight.

Preheat the grill to medium-high heat. Remove the lamb loins and allow them to reach room temperature. When the grill is hot, put the lamb over direct high heat and cook for 2 minutes. Roll the loins a quarter turn and cook for another minute. Repeat this process until all sides are cooked. The internal temperature should be about 130°F (54°C) for medium-rare, 135°F (57°C) for medium, 145°F (63°C) for medium-well, and 150°F (66°C) for well. Remove and allow to rest for 10 minutes before slicing.

YIELD: 2 SERVINGS

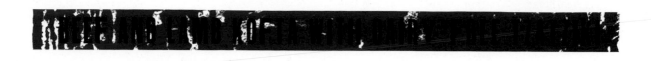

FOR KOFTA:

5 cloves garlic, minced

1 tablespoon (18 g) coarse sea salt

$^1/_2$ pound (227 g) ground chuck

$^1/_2$ pound (227 g) ground lamb

1 medium onion, minced

$^1/_4$ cup (15 g) chopped fresh parsley

1 tablespoon (6 g) ground coriander

1 teaspoon ground cumin

$^1/_2$ teaspoon allspice

$^1/_4$ teaspoon cayenne pepper

Pinch of cinnamon

FOR TZATZIKI SAUCE:

1 cup (240 g) Dairy-free Coconut Sour Cream (page 46)

1 medium cucumber, peeled, seeded, and grated

1 tablespoon (15 ml) extra virgin olive oil

1 teaspoon fresh lemon juice

1 head Bibb lettuce

UNLIKE TYPICAL KEBABS THAT ARE MADE WITH WHOLE SKEWERED PIECES OF MEAT, KOFTA IS GROUND MEAT THAT IS PRESSED AROUND A SKEWER AND GRILLED. THIS RECIPE ALSO INCLUDES A PALEO-FIED VERSION OF THE TRADITIONAL YOGURT-BASED TZATZIKI SAUCE.

TO MAKE THE KOFTA: Soak 14 wooden skewers in water to cover for 30 minutes (or use metal skewers). Using a mortar and pestle make a paste out of the minced garlic and sea salt. Reserve a small amount (1 to 2 teaspoons) for the tzatziki sauce. Combine the garlic paste with all the other kofta ingredients in a large mixing bowl. Cover the bowl and let the meat mixture chill for at least an hour to let the flavors develop (even better if left overnight).

TO MAKE THE TZATZIKI SAUCE: Mix the reserved garlic paste, sour cream, cucumber, olive oil, and lemon juice in a bowl. Put the tzatziki in the refrigerator until ready to serve.

Prepare your grill with a chimney full of coals. Press the meat mixture around the 14 skewers in a long oval shape, leaving at least 2 inches (5 cm) of the skewer exposed on one end. Grill the kofta over direct heat, cooking for 5 minutes before flipping. Cook for an additional 5 minutes. If your grill can't hold all of the kofta at once, work in batches, wrapping finished kebabs in foil to keep them hot.

Serve the kofta with Bibb lettuce leaves and top with the tzatziki.

YIELD: 14 KEBABS

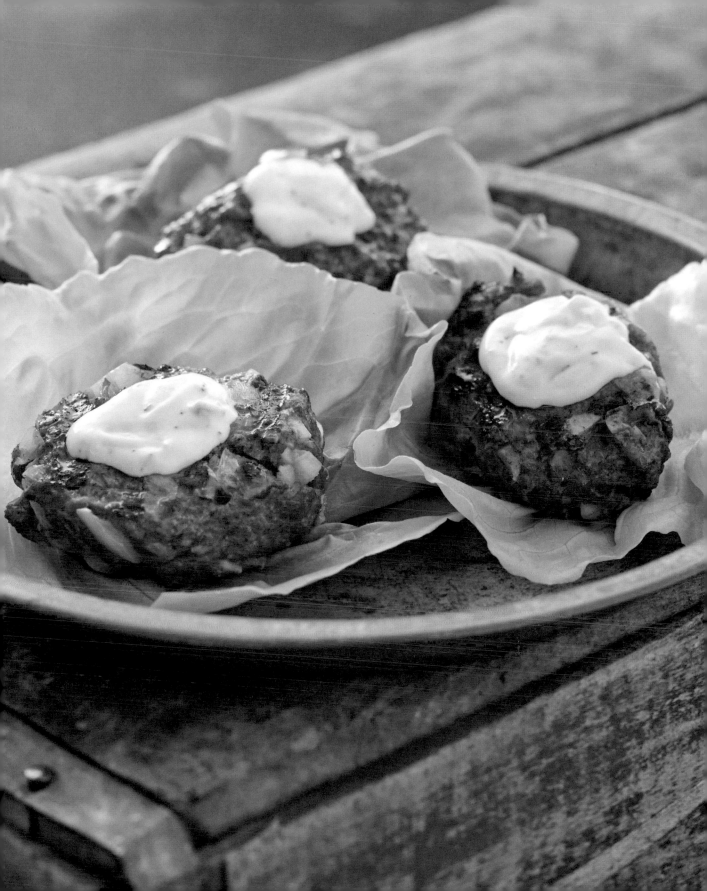

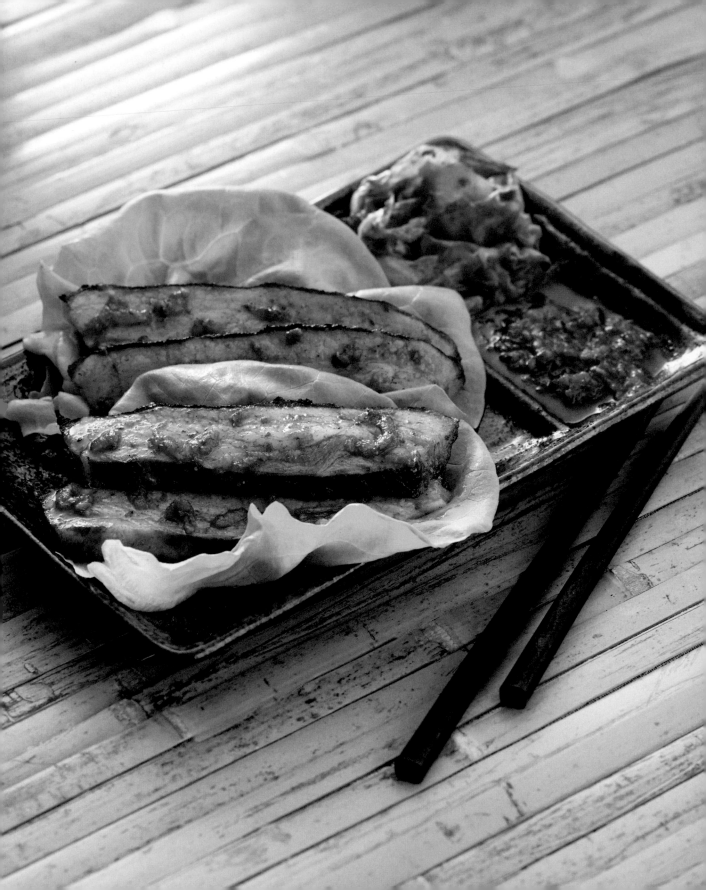

PORK

2¹/₂ pounds (1.1 kg) pork belly in one rectangular piece

2 cups (475 ml) Asian Pear BBQ Marinade (page 52)

1 head Bibb or iceberg lettuce

4 tablespoons (24 g) chopped scallions

2 cups (470 g) kimchi

KOREAN GRILLED PORK BELLY LETTUCE WRAPS

PORK BELLY, THE CUT OF PORK USED TO MAKE BACON, IS PERFECT FOR GRILLING BECAUSE OF ITS ABUNDANT FAT CONTENT. PAIRING GRILLED SWEET AND SPICY MARINATED PORK BELLY WITH THE FLAVOR OF PICKLED KIMCHI CUTS THE GREASINESS, WHILE FRESH LETTUCE CUPS CLEANSE THE PALATE AND MAKE THEM PERFECT FOR ONE-HANDED EATING.

In a glass baking dish, cover the pork belly with the marinade, ensuring that the meat is completely coated. Cover with plastic wrap and allow to marinate overnight in the refrigerator.

Remove the pork belly from the marinade and allow excess marinade to drain off. Preheat the grill to medium heat and cook the pork belly over direct heat for about 10 minutes. Turn the meat often to avoid burning because the high fat and honey may cause flare-ups. Remove the pork belly from the grill and place on paper towels to drain. When cool, cut into 1-inch (2.5 cm) pieces.

Pull apart the lettuce leaves and place as cups. Fill individual lettuce cups with a few pieces of pork belly and garnish with sliced scallion and kimchi.

YIELD: 10 TO 12 SERVINGS

"If I had to narrow my choice of meats down to one for the rest of my life, I am quite certain that meat would be pork." —**JAMES BEARD**

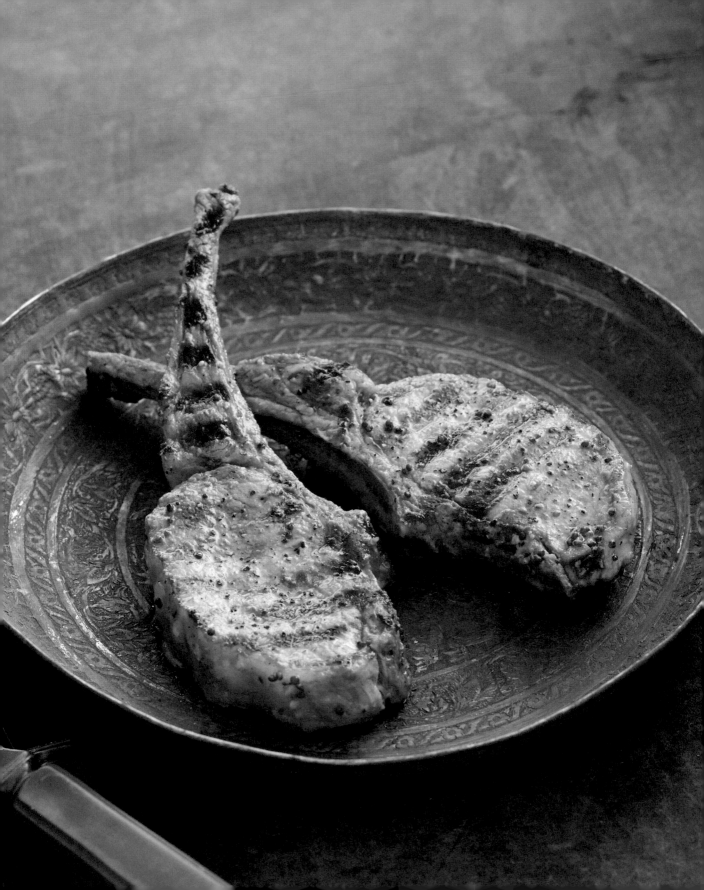

PORK CHOPS SCOTTA DITTA

FOR MARINADE:

¹/₄ cup (44 g) whole-grain mustard

¹/₃ cup (80 ml) Champagne vinegar

2 teaspoons (6 g) minced garlic

¹/₃ cup (55 g) diced red onion

1 cup (235 ml) extra virgin olive oil

¹/₄ cup (10 g) rolled and thinly sliced fresh basil (chiffonade)

¹/₄ cup (16 g) thinly sliced fresh Greek oregano

2 teaspoons (12 g) sea salt

2 teaspoons (4 g) coarsely ground black pepper

FOR CHOPS:

4 bone-in pork loin chops, frenched

THE PHRASE *SCOTTA DITTA* IS ITALIAN FOR "BURNING FINGERS," AND THAT IS WHAT THE BONES IN THESE PORK CHOPS WILL RESEMBLE WHEN FINISHED. TO FRENCH THE PORK CHOPS, USE A SHARP KNIFE TO CUT THE MEAT AWAY FROM THE END OF THE CHOP, EXPOSING THE BONE.

TO MAKE THE MARINADE: Combine all of the marinade ingredients in a glass container with a tight-fitting screw-on lid. Shake the glass jar for 10 seconds and pour one-fourth of it into a medium-size glass baking dish. Place the pork chops in the dish and pour two-thirds of the remaining marinade over the top, reserving the last of the marinade for basting later. Cover the dish with plastic wrap and marinate in the refrigerator for 2 hours.

TO MAKE THE CHOPS: Preheat the grill to high on one side and medium-low on another. Remove the chops from the marinade, and discard the marinade. Place the chops over high heat and grill for 1 minute, turn 90 degrees, and grill for another 1 minute. Flip the chops and repeat on the other side. The outside of the chops should have black grill marks and the bones should start to char.

Move the chops to the lower temperature side of the grill and baste with the reserved marinade. Let cook over low heat with the lid on, turning and basting every couple of minutes. The pork chops are done when they reach an internal temperature of 160°F (71°C).

YIELD: 4 SERVINGS

GRILLED PORK CUTLETS WITH APPLE SAFFRON COMPOTE

FOR APPLE SAFFRON COMPOTE:

3 tablespoons (45 ml) honey

$^1/_2$ cup (120 ml) apple cider vinegar

10 saffron threads

2 Golden Delicious apples, peeled, cored, and diced

FOR CUTLETS:

2 pork tenderloins, trimmed of all fat and silver skin

1 tablespoon (18 g) sea salt

1 tablespoon (6 g) black pepper

2 tablespoons (30 ml) olive oil

THIS IS ONE OF THE MORE INVOLVED RECIPES IN THE BOOK, BUT ITS INDIVIDUAL STEPS ARE SIMPLE. THE TENDER PORK WORKS VERY WELL WITH THE SWEET AND SOUR APPLE SAFFRON COMPOTE.

TO MAKE THE COMPOTE: In a small saucepot over low heat, combine the honey, vinegar, and saffron. Reduce by half until slightly syrupy. This should take about 2 minutes. Add the apples and cook for 2 minutes while stirring. Set aside and allow to cool.

TO MAKE THE CUTLETS: On a clean cutting board, cut the tenderloin into $1^1/_2$-inch (3.8 cm) pieces. With a meat mallet, on that same cutting board, pound the tenderloin gently and evenly until it doubles in diameter. Pieces should be about $^1/_2$ inch (1.3 cm) thick. Place the cutlets on a baking sheet lined with foil and set aside as you prepare the grill.

Season the pork cutlets with salt and pepper. Preheat the grill to medium and lubricate with oil. Put the tenderloin pieces on the grill and cook for 2 minutes. Turn the tenderloin 90 degrees and cook for another 2 minutes. Flip the meat and repeat the process on the other side. When done, the cutlets should have an internal temperature of 134ºF (57ºC). Remove from the grill and let rest for 5 minutes. Top with the compote before serving.

YIELD: 6 TO 8 SERVINGS

SPICY CASHEW PORK KABOBS

FOR SPICY CASHEW MARINADE:

¼ cup (60 ml) red wine vinegar

3 tablespoons (45 ml) full-fat coconut milk

2 tablespoons (28 g) coconut oil, melted

1½ teaspoons sesame oil

Zest and juice of 1 lime

2 tablespoons (30 g) cashew butter

1 teaspoon black sesame seeds

1 tablespoon (6 g) minced ginger

1 tablespoon (1 g) roughly chopped fresh cilantro

2 teaspoons (6 g) minced garlic

½ teaspoon red pepper flakes

FOR PORK:

1½ pounds (680 g) pork loin, trimmed of all fat and cut into 1-inch (2.5 cm) cubes

MARINATING LEAN PORK LOIN AND COOKING IT QUICKLY OVER HIGH HEAT ENSURES THAT THE MEAT STAYS MOIST. ALTHOUGH THE PALEO DIET DOESN'T ADVOCATE COUNTING CALORIES, THIS IS CERTAINLY A LOWER-CALORIE RECIPE THAT STILL TASTES INDULGENT.

TO MAKE THE MARINADE: Combine the vinegar, coconut milk, coconut oil, sesame oil, lime juice, and cashew butter in a mixing bowl. Whisk gently at first and more aggressively as the mixture becomes smoother. When the mixture is smooth, add the sesame seeds, ginger, cilantro, garlic, red pepper flakes, and lime zest.

TO MAKE THE PORK: Place the pork loin and marinade into a zip-top bag. Ensure that the meat is completely coated and then place in the refrigerator to marinate for 6 to 8 hours.

Remove the pork from the marinade and drain thoroughly. Using metal skewers, thread 5 or 6 cubes of pork onto each skewer. Let sit at room temperature for 20 to 30 minutes.

Oil and preheat your grill to medium-high heat. Place the kabobs on the grill and cook for approximately 15 minutes, or until the internal temperature reaches 150°F (66°C).

YIELD: 8 TO 10 SERVINGS

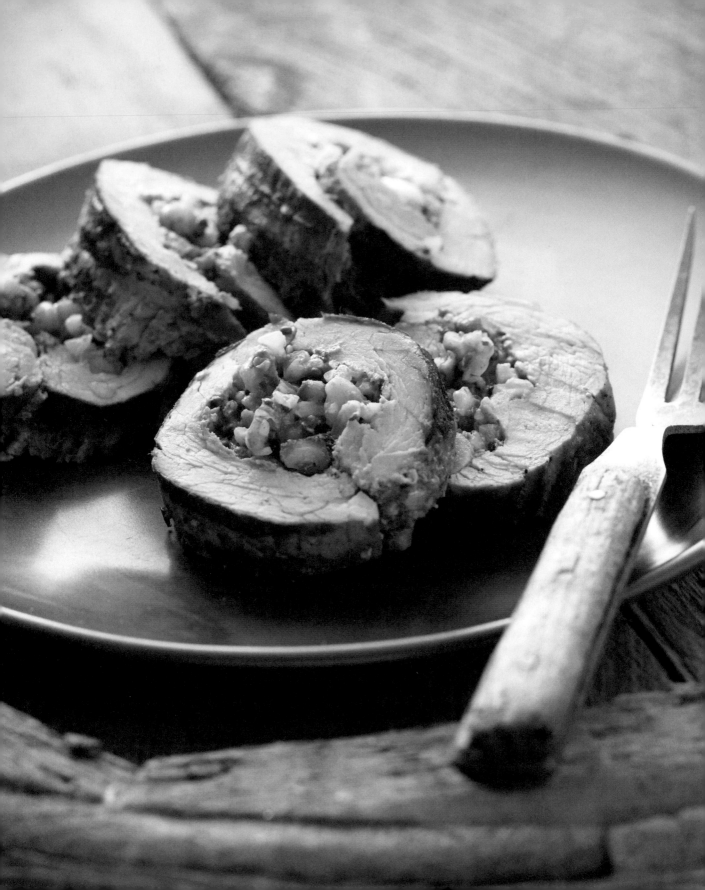

PORK TENDERLOIN ROULADE

FOR STUFFING:

1 shallot, minced

3 tablespoons (30 g) walnuts, toasted and crushed

1 tablespoon (11 g) whole-grain mustard

$1/2$ teaspoon honey

2 tablespoons (2.5 g) chopped fresh thyme, stems removed

FOR ROULADE:

1 pound (454 g) pork tenderloin, trimmed of silver skin and excess fat

Baker's twine soaked in water, cut into four 5-inch (12.5 cm) pieces

Kosher salt and black pepper

Olive oil

BY STUFFING THE LEAN PORK TENDERLOIN WITH A MIXTURE OF NUTS, HERBS, AND SPICES, YOU NOT ONLY ADD FLAVOR TO THE DISH, BUT YOU ALSO GET A REFINED PRESENTATION THAT IS PERFECT FOR IMPRESSING GUESTS.

TO MAKE THE STUFFING: In a small bowl, combine the shallots, walnuts, mustard, honey, and thyme. With gloves on, work the mixture thoroughly with your hands. It should form a thick paste.

TO MAKE THE ROULADE: Prepare the grill to medium heat. Using a sharp knife, cut the tenderloin lengthwise about halfway through. Be careful not to cut it too much. Open up the tenderloin and loosely cover it with plastic wrap. Using a meat mallet or the bottom of a heavy skillet, pound the tenderloin until it is uniformly $1/4$ inch (6 mm) thick.

Smear the walnut paste evenly on the inside portion of the tenderloin, leaving a $1/4$ inch (6 mm) border on all sides. Gently roll the tenderloin. Tie the four pieces of twine around the tenderloin using just enough pressure to keep it together. Season the outside of the roulade with salt and pepper. Rub a small amount of olive oil on the outside of the roulade. Place on the grill over direct heat. Roll it one-third every 8 to 10 minutes until it is cooked on all sides and has an internal temperature of 155°F (68°C). Remove from the grill and let rest for 10 minutes. Cut the roulade into 8 even portions.

YIELD: 8 SERVINGS

SALT-CURED APPLEWOOD-SMOKED BACON

1 cup (288 g) sea salt

¹/₂ cup (100 g) coconut sugar

4 tablespoons (24 g) ground black pepper

1 tablespoon (4 g) ground thyme (optional)

1 tablespoon (2 g) ground rosemary (optional)

3 to 5 pounds (1.4 to 2.3 kg) pastured pork belly

1 pound (453 g) applewood chunks (preferred) or chips

Aluminum pan and hot water (optional)

Aluminum foil (if using wood chips without a smoker box)

BACON IS A KEY INGREDIENT IN MANY RECIPES BECAUSE EVEN A SMALL AMOUNT ADDS A TON OF FLAVOR. BACON CAN BE PRICY, BUT YOU CAN MAKE IT AT HOME FOR ABOUT HALF THE COST. THIS RECIPE MAKES USE OF A GAS OR CHARCOAL GRILL, BUT YOU CAN DEFINITELY USE A DEDICATED SMOKER AS WELL.

Make a curing mixture by combine the sea salt, coconut sugar, black pepper, and herbs in a bowl. Thoroughly rub the pork belly with the curing mix, ensuring that all sides are thickly coated. Reserve the remaining curing mixture. Put the pork belly into a large zip-top bag and put in the refrigerator. Allow the pork belly to cure for 1 week, flipping the bag daily. Remove the pork belly from the bag and rub it with fresh curing mixture. Put the pork belly into a new zip-top bag and allow it to cure for 1 more week in the refrigerator.

When the pork belly has properly cured, remove it from the bag and completely rinse off all the curing mix. Pat the pork belly dry, put it on a plate, and refrigerate overnight to dry further.

Prepare your grill (see "Smoking Without a Smoker" on page 31) and place about 2 ounces (56 g) of wood chunks/chips on top of the hot coals. For a gas grill, you can simply add the wood chips to your smoker box and place directly over a burner on one side.

Put the meat on the side of the grill receiving indirect heat (over the water pan if you are using one) and close the lid of the grill. As the meat cooks, adjust the intake damper vents to keep the temperature of the grill around the meat close to 225°F (107°C). Add about 6 hot coals and 2 ounces (56 g) of wood every 30 minutes or so to maintain the temperature. Cracking the lid of the grill, or adding an additional pan full of water to the top grate, can help if the temperature is running too hot. Cooking time should run about 90 minutes per pound (450 g) and the meat is done when it reaches an internal temperature of 160°F (71°C).

Allow the bacon to cool before slicing. The bacon should keep for about a week refrigerated.

YIELD: 6 SERVINGS

GRILLED PORK JOWLS WITH PEPPERS AND ONIONS

1 pound (455 g) smoked pork jowl, cut into 3-ounce (85 g) lengthwise slices (like thick-cut bacon)

1 green bell pepper, cut in half, seeded, and cored

1 red bell pepper, cut in half, seeded, and cored

1 red onion, cut into thick rings

1 Anaheim chile

1 Roma tomato

2 tablespoons (30 ml) olive oil

1 teaspoon minced garlic

1 teaspoon sambal or sriracha chili sauce

10 to 12 fresh cilantro leaves

PORK JOWL IS SIMILAR TO BACON BUT OFTEN CHEAPER AND MORE FLAVORFUL. LIKE BACON, IT IS OFTEN USED TO FLAVOR OTHER DISHES, BUT IN THIS PARTICULAR RECIPE, THE JOWL IS THE STAR.

Preheat the grill to high. Place the jowl on the rack above the grill. Put the lid on the grill and cook for 1 minute, until the fat from the jowl starts to render. Place the vegetables directly below the pork jowl so the fat dripping from the jowl flavors the vegetables. Close the lid again and cook for 1 minute.

Working quickly with long tongs, open the grill and flip the vegetables and jowl. Replace the lid on the grill and cook for 1 more minute. Remove the vegetables from the grill and place on a baking sheet to cool. Continue to cook the jowl for 5 to 10 minutes, until it has achieved the desired doneness. The fat should be rendered and the jowl slices will be golden brown.

When the vegetables have cooled enough to handle, cut into strips and place in a mixing bowl. Add the olive oil, garlic, and sambal and toss to coat thoroughly. Cut the jowl into bite-size chunks and serve with the grilled vegetables. Garnish with the cilantro leaves.

YIELD: 4 SERVINGS

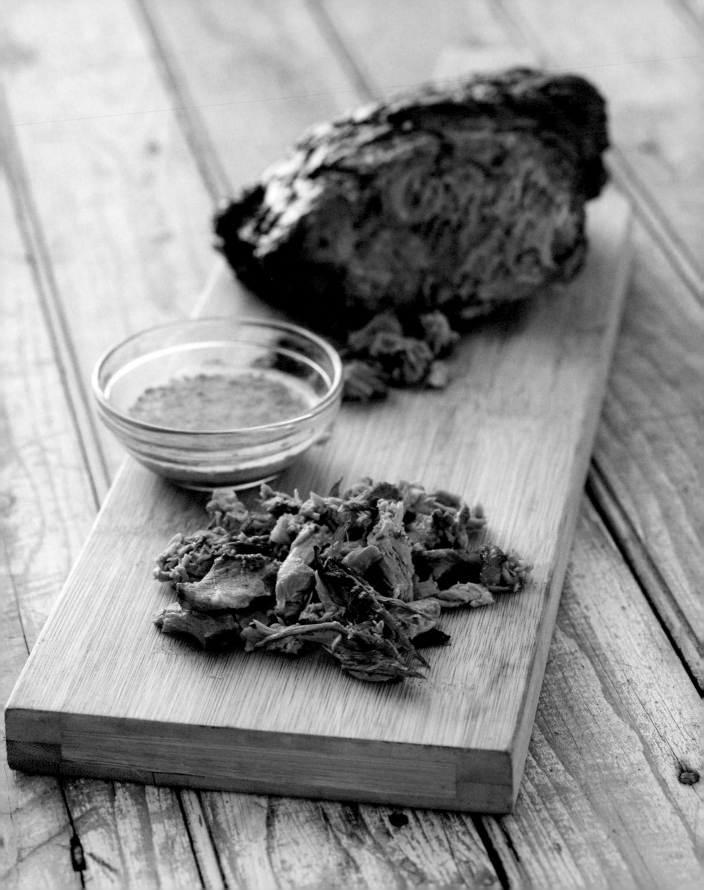

MOJO PORK SHOULDER

FOR MOJO MARINADE:

5 cups (1.2 L) orange juice

1 cup (235 ml) lime juice

Zest of 1 lime

Zest of 1 orange

10 to 12 cloves garlic, roughly chopped

1 yellow onion, roughly chopped

1 teaspoon coriander seeds

Sea salt and coarsely ground black pepper

2 ounces (56 g) chopped fresh Cuban or Mexican oregano

FOR PORK:

1 bone-in pork shoulder (4 to 5 pounds [1.8 to 2.3 kg])

Aluminum pan and hot water (optional)

THERE ARE MANY TYPES OF MOJOS FROM MANY DIFFERENT PLACES. ORIGINALLY A PORTUGUESE SAUCE, IT IS NOW CLAIMED BY PEOPLE IN ALL OF THE CARIBBEAN AND SOUTHERN UNITED STATES AS FAR NORTH AS NORTH CAROLINA. THIS RECIPE IS DESIGNED TO GIVE YOU "FALL OFF THE BONE" TENDERNESS EVEN WHEN USING A STANDARD GRILL.

TO MAKE THE MARINADE: Combine all of the marinade ingredients except the oregano in a large pot. Heat over medium heat until it barely simmers, then remove from the heat. Allow to cool completely, and then add the oregano.

TO MAKE THE PORK: Score the skin of the pork shoulder using a crosshatch pattern, cutting through the fat to the flesh. Place the pork shoulder in a glass dish. Reserve 1 cup (235 ml) of the marinade and pour the rest over the pork shoulder, cover in plastic wrap, and allow to marinate in the refrigerator for at least 4 hours and as long as overnight.

When ready to cook, remove the shoulder from the marinade and let it sit at room temperature for 30 minutes. Prepare your grill as if you were going to smoke the pork (see "Smoking Without a Smoker" on page 31). Put the meat on the side of the grill receiving indirect heat (over the water pan if you are using one) and close the lid of the grill.

As the meat cooks, adjust the intake damper vents to keep the temperature of the grill around the meat as close to 225°F (107°C) as you can. You may need to also add more coals to keep the temperature up. Add about 6 hot coals every 30 minutes or so to maintain the temperature. Cracking the lid of the grill, or adding an additional pan full of water to the top grate, can also help if the temperature is running too hot. Cooking time should run about 90 minutes per pound (450 g) and the meat is done when it reaches an internal temperature of 160°F (71°C).

While the pork shoulder is still hot, use two forks to shred the pork. Mix the shredded pork with the reserved marinade and serve.

YIELD: 8 TO 10 SERVINGS

GRILLED PORK RIBS WITH CHERRY GASTRIQUE

FOR RIBS:

3-pound (1.4 kg) slab pork back ribs

¼ cup (28 g) Rib Rub (page 48)

Aluminum foil

Aluminum pan and hot water (optional)

FOR CHERRY GASTRIQUE:

3 tablespoons (60 g) honey

½ cup (120 ml) Champagne vinegar

20 to 25 fresh cherries, stemmed, cut in half, and pitted

RIBS CAN BE TRICKY. YOU WANT THE MEAT TO BE PROPERLY CARAMELIZED, BUT YOU DON'T WANT IT TO GET TOUGH. ALLOWING THE RIBS TO COOK MOST OF THE WAY ENCASED IN FOIL AND FINISHING DIRECTLY ON THE GRILL ENSURES THAT THE RIBS WILL BE PROPERLY SLOW COOKED AND STILL ACHIEVE A NICE GOLDEN BROWN CRUST.

TO MAKE THE RIBS: Cover the ribs liberally with the rub and wrap loosely in aluminum foil, making sure the edges are tightly sealed.

Prepare your grill as if you were going to smoke the ribs (see "Smoking Without a Smoker" on page 31). Put the meat on the side of the grill receiving indirect heat (over the water pan if you are using one) and close the lid of the grill.

As the meat cooks, adjust the intake damper vents to keep the temperature of the grill around the meat as close to 225°F (107°C) as you can. You may need to also add more coals to keep the temperature up. Add about 6 hot coals every 30 minutes or so to maintain the temperature. Cracking the lid of the grill, or adding an additional pan full of water to the top grate, can also help if the temperature is running too hot. Total cooking time should run about 90 minutes per pound (450 g), so a 3 pound (1.4 kg) slab should take about 4 hours. At the three hour mark, remove the ribs from the foil and reserve the juice. Cook the ribs for the remainder of the time uncovered, turning the ribs every 15 minutes and basting with the reserved juices until done.

When finished, the internal temperature of the meat should be 160°F (71°C) and the rib bones should pull away easily.

TO MAKE THE GASTRIQUE: Combine the honey and vinegar in a small saucepot. Heat over medium heat until reduced by half. This should take about 2 minutes. Add the cherries and simmer for 2 minutes. Remove from the heat and allow to cool to room temperature.

Top the ribs with gastrique before serving.

YIELD: 6 TO 8 SERVINGS

SMOKED PORK TENDERLOIN WITH BACON MUSTARD VINAIGRETTE

FOR TENDERLOIN:

2 pieces (1 pound, or 454 g, each) pork tenderloin

1 quart (940 ml) Sweet and Savory Spice Brine (page 53)

2 cups (470 ml) apple cider vinegar

1 pound (453g) applewood chunks (preferred) or chips

Aluminum pan and hot water (optional)

Aluminum foil (if using wood chips without a smoker box)

Black pepper

FOR BACON MUSTARD VINAIGRETTE:

¹/₂ pound (227 g) bacon

1 medium Spanish onion, diced

1 tablespoon (10 g) minced garlic

2 tablespoons (30 ml) maple syrup

¹/₂ cup (120 ml) apple cider vinegar

2 tablespoons (22 g) whole-grain mustard

1 tablespoon (2.5 g) fresh thyme

Black pepper

PORK TENDERLOIN IS TYPICALLY LEAN AND CAN EASILY BECOME TOUGH AND DRY IF YOU AREN'T CAREFUL. BRINING THE TENDERLOIN BEFORE SMOKING HELPS THE MEAT RETAIN MORE MOISTURE, KEEPING IT TENDER AND JUICY IN ADDITION TO INFUSING THE MEAT WITH MORE FLAVOR.

TO MAKE THE TENDERLOIN: Trim the pork tenderloin, removing all the silver skin. Place in a plastic container with at least 4-inch (10 cm) sides and pour the spice brine and apple cider vinegar over the tenderloins, submerging completely. Allow to marinate in the brine in the refrigerator overnight. When ready to cook, remove the tenderloins from the brine, pat dry, and season with freshly cracked black pepper.

Prepare your grill for smoking (see "Smoking Without a Smoker" on page 31) and add about 2 ounces (56 g) of wood chunks/chips on top of the hot coals. For a gas grill, you can simply add the wood chips to your smoker box and place directly over a burner on one side. Put the meat on the side of the grill receiving direct heat (opposite the water pan if you are using one) and sear for approximately 2 minutes per side. After the tenderloin is seared, move it to the side of the grill receiving indirect heat and close the lid of the grill.

As the meat cooks, adjust the intake damper vents to keep the temperature of the grill close to 225°F (107°C). You may need to add more coals to keep the temperature up. Add about 6 hot coals and 2 ounces (56 g) of wood every 30 minutes or so to maintain the temperature. Cracking the lid of the grill, or adding an additional pan full of water to the top grate, can also help if the grill is running too hot. Cooking time should run about 90 minutes per pound (450 g) and the meat is done when it reaches an internal temperature of 150°F (65°C).

When the tenderloins are done, remove them from the grill and allow to rest covered for 5–10 minutes before slicing. Top with the bacon mustard vinaigrette before serving.

TO MAKE THE VINAIGRETTE: Cut the bacon into thin ribbons. Render in a hot pan until slightly crispy. Without draining the bacon fat, add the onion and garlic. Stir while cooking until the onions are tender. Stir in the maple syrup, apple cider vinegar, mustard, thyme, and pepper and simmer for 2 minutes. Turn off the heat and set aside.

YIELD: 4 SERVINGS

HOUSE-MADE SMOKED ANDOUILLE SAUSAGE

**5 pounds (2.3 kg)
boneless pork butt**

8 ounces (227 g) pork fat

²/₃ cup (100 g) chopped garlic

¹/₄ cup (24 g) black pepper

**2 tablespoons (10 g)
cayenne pepper**

**2 tablespoons (14 g)
sweet paprika**

2 tablespoons (8 g) dried thyme

2 tablespoons (36 g) salt

6 feet (1.8 m) beef middle casing

**1 pound (453g) hickory, oak, or
pecan chunks (preferred) or chips**

**Aluminum pan and hot water
(optional)**

**Aluminum foil (if using wood
chips without a smoker box)**

THERE ARE FEW THINGS MORE SATISFYING THAN MAKING SAUSAGE. THERE ARE UNLIMITED NUMBERS OF FLAVORS AND TEXTURES THAT YOU CAN COMBINE, SO HOPEFULLY DOING IT ONCE WILL GIVE YOU THE CONFIDENCE TO TRY OTHER RECIPES IN THE FUTURE.

Cut the pork butt and fat into 1-inch (2.5 cm) cubes. Cover and return the meat to the refrigerator for 1 hour to chill. Using a meat grinder with four ¼-inch (6 mm) holes in the grinding plate, grind the pork and fat, alternating between the two. Place the ground pork in a large mixing bowl and, working quickly, incorporate the seasonings.

Once well blended, use the sausage attachment on your meat grinder to stuff the sausage casing. Start by tying one end of the casing with butcher's twine. Turn on the grinder and extrude the ground meat into the casing in a smooth, continuous motion, pulling the sausage forward and turning the sausage in a circle. When all of the meat is encased, push the meat forward in the casing and cut the remaining casing, leaving 1 ½ inches (3.8 cm) of casing from the sausage. Tie that end tightly with butcher's twine. Estimate about 5 inches (12.5 cm) in length from the end of the sausage rope, pinch it, and twist the sausage toward you 4 times. Moving down the length of the sausage, estimate another 5 inch length (12.5 cm), pinch it, and twist it away from you 4 times. Repeat this until the entire rope is divided into links.

Prepare your grill for smoking (see "Smoking Without a Smoker" on page 31) and add about 2 ounces (56 g) of wood chunks/chips on top of the hot coals. For a gas grill, you can simply add the wood chips to your smoker box and place directly over a burner on one side.

Put the meat on the side of the grill receiving indirect heat (over the water pan if you are using one) and close the lid of the grill. As the meat cooks, adjust the intake damper vents to keep the temperature of the grill around the meat as close to 225°F (107°C) as you can. You may need to also add more coals to keep the temperature up. Add about 6 hot coals and 2 ounces (56 g) of wood every 30 minutes or so to maintain the temperature. Cracking the lid of the grill, or adding an additional pan full of water to the top grate, can also help if the temperature is running too hot. Cooking time should run about 90 minutes per pound (450 g) and the meat is done when it reaches an internal temperature of 160°F (71°C).

YIELD: 12 TO 14 SAUSAGES

NORTH CAROLINA PORK BARBECUE WITH COUNTRY SLAW

1 pound (453g) hickory, oak, or pecan chunks (preferred) or chips

Aluminum pan and hot water (optional)

Aluminum foil (if using wood chips without a smoker box)

6-pound (2.7 kg) Boston butt

2 cups (475 ml) Tangy Vinegar Moppin' Sauce (page 45)

2 cups (150 g) Crisp Country Slaw (page 65), for serving

IN NORTH CAROLINA, PIG IS THE KING OF THE BARBECUE PIT. SLOW COOKED UNTIL FORK-TENDER, IT IS SERVED EVERYWHERE FROM CORNER STORES TO CHURCH PICNICS. TRADITIONALLY DONE IN A SMOKER, THIS RECIPE HAS BEEN MODIFIED TO GIVE YOU GREAT RESULTS WITH A STANDARD BACKYARD GRILL.

Prepare your grill for smoking (see "Smoking Without a Smoker" on page 31) and add about 2 ounces (56 g) of wood chunks/chips on top of the hot coals. For a gas grill, you can simply add the wood chips to your smoker box and place directly over a burner on one side.

Put the meat on the side of the grill receiving indirect heat (over the water pan if you are using one) and close the lid of the grill. As the meat cooks, adjust the intake damper vents to keep the temperature of the grill around the meat as close to 225°F (107°C) as you can. You may need to also add more coals to keep the temperature up. Add about 6 hot coals and 2 ounces (56 g) of wood every 30 minutes or so to maintain the temperature. Cracking the lid of the grill, or adding an additional pan full of water to the top grate, can also help if the temperature is running too hot.

Cooking time should run about 9 hours (90 minutes per pound [450 g]), so halfway through the cooking time, wrap the pork butt in foil. This will help prevent the meat from drying out. At this point, if you are having trouble keeping the temperature of the grill constant, you could also finish the pork butt in an oven heated to 225°F (107°C). The meat is done when it reaches an internal temperature of 160°F (71°C).

Let the pork butt sit wrapped in foil for 30 minutes before pulling. Using gloves and tongs, shred the meat and dress it with sauce while still hot. Serve with Crisp Country Slaw.

YIELD: 10 TO 12 SERVINGS

SMOKED PORK SHANKS

2 pork shanks, 1¹/₂ pounds (680 g) each

4 tablespoons (28 g) Pig Rub (page 48)

1 pound (453g) hickory, oak, or pecan chunks (preferred) or chips

Aluminum pan and hot water (optional)

Aluminum foil (if using wood chips without a smoker box)

PORK SHANKS USED TO BE HARD TO FIND BUT ARE READILY AVAILABLE NOW THAT PEOPLE HAVE CAUGHT ON TO THIS CUT. IT'S A CHEAP ITEM THAT, WHEN PROPERLY PREPARED, WILL YIELD A SUCCULENT AND SAVORY ROUNDED FLAVOR. THESE ARE DELICIOUS SERVED WITH BACON YAM SALAD (PAGE 65).

Coat the shanks thoroughly with the rub and refrigerate for 2 hours. When ready to cook, put the shanks on a platter and allow them to come to room temperature.

Prepare your grill for smoking (see "Smoking Without a Smoker" on page 31) and add about 2 ounces (56 g) of wood chunks on top of the hot coals. For a gas grill, you can simply add the wood chips to your smoker box and place directly over a burner on one side.

Put the meat on the side of the grill receiving indirect heat (over the water pan if you are using one) and close the lid of the grill. As the meat cooks, adjust the intake damper vents to keep the temperature of the grill around the meat as close to 225°F (107°C) as you can. You may need to also add more coals to keep the temperature up. Add about 6 hot coals and 2 ounces (56 g) of wood every 30 minutes or so to maintain the temperature. Cracking the lid of the grill, or adding an additional pan full of water to the top grate, can also help if the temperature is running too hot. Cooking time should run about 90 minutes per pound (450 g) and the meat is done when it reaches an internal temperature of 160°F (71°C).

YIELD: 2 TO 4 SERVINGS

THE PICKLED PORKER

FOR PICKLED RED ONIONS:

1 1/2 cups (355 ml) red wine vinegar

2 tablespoons (25 g) coconut sugar

1 red onion, cut in half and thinly sliced

FOR ROASTED GREEN CHILES:

1 medium poblano chile

2 Hatch or Anaheim chiles

1 serrano chile

1/4 cup (60 ml) red wine vinegar

1 tablespoon (15 ml) extra virgin olive oil

3 tablespoons (3 g) fresh cilantro

Kosher salt and black pepper

FOR PORK:

1 1/2 pounds (680 g) 80/20 ground pork

Kosher salt and black pepper

BEEF TENDS TO GET ALL THE BURGER LOVE, BUT GROUND PORK IS A PERFECTLY VIABLE BURGER BASE, TOO. IN THIS RECIPE, THE FLAVOR OF PORK COMBINED WITH ROASTED GREEN CHILES AND PICKLED RED ONIONS WILL MAKE YOU FORGET TO ASK, "WHERE'S THE BEEF?"

TO MAKE THE PICKLED ONIONS: Heat the vinegar and coconut sugar in a small saucepot over medium heat until the mixture simmers. Turn off the heat and whisk until the coconut sugar is completely dissolved. While still warm, pour over the onions in a bowl. Refrigerate, uncovered, until cool.

TO MAKE THE CHILES: Preheat a grill to high heat. Place all of the chiles on the grill over direct heat. Grill, rotating with tongs, until the skins are completely black. This should take 8 to 10 minutes. Using tongs, transfer the chiles to a plastic container and wrap tightly with plastic wrap. In 30 minutes, remove the plastic wrap. Using a dry towel, rub away all of the skins from the chiles. Cut open the chiles with a paring knife and remove the stems and seeds. Add the chiles, red wine vinegar, extra virgin olive oil, cilantro, and salt and pepper to taste to a food processor. Pulse until fully incorporated but still chunky. This should take about 20 pulses.

TO MAKE THE PORK: Lower the grill to medium heat. Divide the ground pork into 6 portions and form into burgers. Season with salt and black pepper. Grill for 4 minutes on each side with the lid on. Transfer to the rack over the grill and allow to finish if not done enough. When the burgers are done, remove from the grill and top with the chiles and pickled onions.

YIELD: 6 SERVINGS

GLAZED GINGER PEACH STUFFED PORK LOIN

FOR GINGER PEACH STUFFING:

2 tablespoons (28 g) coconut oil

2 shallots, sliced

1-inch (2.5 cm) piece ginger, minced

2 cloves garlic, minced

4 ripe peaches, pitted and sliced

1 dried chipotle pepper, soaked in hot water and chopped

1 tablespoon (20 g) raw organic honey

FOR GLAZE:

1 tablespoon (14 g) coconut oil

2 cloves garlic, minced

$1/2$-inch (1.3 cm) piece ginger, minced

3 ripe peaches, pitted and chopped

1 dried chipotle pepper, soaked in hot water and chopped

3 tablespoons (60 g) raw organic honey

$1/2$ cup (120 ml) apple cider vinegar

Sea salt

SWEET AND CARAMELIZED ON THE OUTSIDE, WITH A SAVORY HEAT ON THE INSIDE, THIS BONELESS GLAZED PORK TENDERLOIN IS A PALEO PARTY IN YOUR MOUTH. THE RECIPE COMES COURTESY OF CRISTINA LIANOS OF HEALTHILINGUIST.COM.

TO MAKE THE STUFFING: Heat the coconut oil in a large sauté pan over medium-low heat until melted. Add the shallots and sauté for 10 minutes, until soft. Add the ginger and garlic and continue sautéing for another 10 minutes. Add the peaches and chipotle peppers and sauté until the peaches are slightly soft, about 5 minutes. Turn off the heat and stir in the honey. Set aside.

TO MAKE THE GLAZE: Heat the coconut oil in a sauté pan over medium-low heat until melted. Add the garlic and ginger and sauté for 2 to 3 minutes, or until soft. Lower the heat and add the peaches, chipotle pepper, honey, and vinegar. Season with sea salt to taste and stir, mashing the peaches. Allow the glaze to reduce for 5 minutes, and then remove from the heat.

FOR PORK:

4-pound (1.8 kg) boneless center-cut pork loin, trimmed and roll cut or butterflied

Sea salt and cracked black pepper

2 teaspoons (4 g) cumin seeds, crushed, divided

1 cup (16 g) chopped cilantro

TO MAKE THE PORK: Preheat the grill to 450ºF (230ºC). Season the cut side of the pork loin with salt, pepper, and 1 teaspoon of the cumin. Arrange the cilantro over the loin and add the ginger peach stuffing, spreading it just shy of the edges. Beginning on one end, roll the loin up, pushing the stuffing in if it seeps out. Secure the rolled-up loin with twine. Turn the loin seam side down, fat side up, and generously sprinkle with salt and the remaining 1 teaspoon cumin.

Sear the loin on the grill, fat side down, for 1 minute. Rotate the loin a quarter turn and repeat until all sides are seared. Lower the grill temperature to 225°F (107°C) and move the loin to indirect heat. Cook for 1¹/₂ to 2 hours, brushing the glaze on for the last 15 to 20 minutes of cooking. The loin is done when it registers an internal temperature of 140°F (60°C). Allow the loin to rest for 10 minutes before slicing.

YIELD: 8 TO 10 SERVINGS

WHY IS THE TENDERLOIN SO TENDER?

What we call the "tenderloin" is actually the pig's psoas muscle. The psoas, used for posture, doesn't get worked out as vigorously as the large muscles of the shoulders, hips, and legs, so it stays nice and soft, perfect for Paleo grilling!

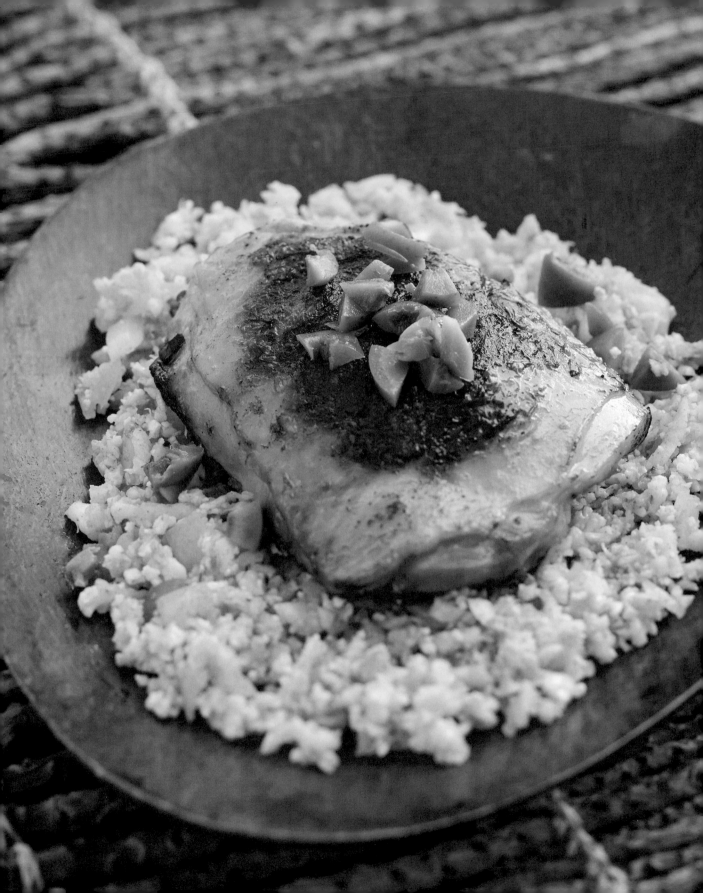

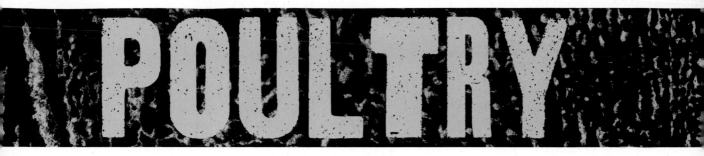
2 pounds (940 g) boneless chicken thighs, trimmed of fat and quartered

2 cups (470 ml) Adobo Marinade (page 52)

1 head cauliflower, core and leaves removed

2 tablespoons (28 g) coconut oil

¹/₄ cup (40 g) chopped yellow onion

2 teaspoons (2 g) powdered saffron or powdered turmeric

2 tablespoons (30 ml) olive oil

10 Castelvetrano olives, pitted (or picholine or manzanilla olives)

CHICKEN ADOBO
WITH SAFFRON CAULIFLOWER RICE

CASTELVETRANO OLIVES HAVE A FRUITY, BUTTERY FLAVOR AND SMOOTH TEXTURE. THEY ARE VERY SMALL AND HAVE A HIGH OIL CONTENT, WHICH LENDS THEM MORE TO OLIVE OIL PRODUCTION THAN TABLE TREAT. OLIVES IN GENERAL ARE AN EXCELLENT BURST OF FLAVOR TO COMPLEMENT JUICY, FATTY CHICKEN THIGHS.

Place the chicken thighs in a large plastic container and pour the marinade over, ensuring they are evenly covered. Cover and marinate in the refrigerator for 8 to 24 hours.

Cut the cauliflower into quarters. Grate it with the coarse side of a box grater or with the grating blade of a food processor.

Heat a large sauté pan over medium-high heat. Add the coconut oil and heat for 15 seconds. Add the onion and sweat for 2 minutes, stirring constantly, until translucent. Add the cauliflower to the pan and sauté for 1 minute, or just until heated through. Add the saffron and stir to combine. Transfer to a serving bowl.

Preheat the grill to medium heat. Remove the chicken thighs from the marinade and discard the marinade. Pat dry with paper towels and rub with the olive oil. Lay the thighs on the grill so that they are evenly spaced. Grill the thighs for 4 to 6 minutes and turn over. Grill another 4 to 6 minutes and poke with a paring knife. If the juices are clear and not pink at all, the thighs are done. Place on top of the saffron cauliflower rice and top with the olives.

YIELD: 6 SERVINGS

"The way you cut your meat reflects the way you live." —**CONFUCIUS**

SMOKED CHICKEN WITH SWISS CHARD, GOLDEN RAISINS, APPLES, AND PINE NUTS

FOR CHICKEN:

3-pound (1.4 kg) chicken, halved

1 gallon (3.7 L) Sweet and Savory Spice Brine (page 53)

¼ pound (113 g) applewood chunks (preferred) or chips

Aluminum pan and hot water (optional)

Aluminum foil (if using wood chips without a smoker box)

Spray bottle filled with half apple juice and half water

FOR SWISS CHARD:

1 tablespoon (15 ml) extra virgin olive oil

1 Granny Smith apple, cored, quartered, and thinly sliced

Juice of 1 lemon

1 pound (454 g) Swiss chard

1 tablespoon (9 g) toasted pine nuts

1 tablespoon (9 g) golden raisins

SINCE CHICKEN LACKS THE COPIOUS FAT OF PORK OR BEEF, A GOOD BRINING HELPS KEEP THE MEAT MOIST. FOR THE BEST FLAVOR, TRY A COMBINATION OF OAK AND APPLEWOOD.

TO PREPARE THE CHICKEN: Rinse the chicken halves thoroughly and place in a large bucket or bowl. Pour the brine over the chicken so that it is completely submerged. Cover the container with plastic wrap and refrigerate for 8 to 24 hours. When ready to cook, place the chicken on a platter and allow to come to room temperature.

Prepare your grill for smoking (see "Smoking Without a Smoker" on page 31) and add about 2 ounces (56 g) of wood chunks/chips on top of the hot coals. For a gas grill, you can simply add the wood chips to your smoker box and place directly over a burner on one side.

Put the meat on the side of the grill receiving indirect heat (over the water pan if you are using one) and close the lid of the grill. As the meat cooks, adjust the intake damper vents to keep the temperature of the grill around the meat as close to 225°F (107°C) as you can. You may need to also add more coals to keep the temperature up. Add about 6 hot coals and 2 ounces (56 g) of wood every 30 minutes or so to maintain the temperature. Cracking the lid of the grill, or adding an additional pan full of water to the top grate, can also help if the temperature is running too hot. Cooking time should run about 90 minutes per pound (450 g) and the meat is done when it reaches an internal temperature of 165°F (73°C).

TO PREPARE THE SWISS CHARD: Heat a large sauté pan with olive oil and when the oil starts to smoke, carefully add the apple, cooking until they turn golden brown, about 5 minutes. Add the lemon juice and then immediately add the Swiss chard, allowing it to wilt while stirring for several minutes. Remove the pan from the heat and stir in the pine nuts and golden raisins.

When ready to serve, place the chicken halves on plates and top with the Swiss chard.

YIELD: 2 TO 4 SERVINGS

MOJO MARINATED CHICKEN BREAST WITH AVOCADO AND PAPAYA SALAD

FOR MOJO MARINADE:

5 cups (1.2 L) orange juice

1 cup (235 ml) lime juice

Zest of 1 lime

Zest of 1 orange

10 to 12 cloves garlic, roughly chopped

1 yellow onion, roughly chopped

1 teaspoon coriander seeds

Sea salt and coarsely ground black pepper

2 ounces (56 g) chopped fresh Cuban or Mexican oregano

FOR CHICKEN:

4 boneless chicken breasts, skin on

FOR AVOCADO AND PAPAYA SALAD:

1 avocado, peeled, pitted, and diced into 1/4-inch (6 mm) cubes

1 papaya, peeled, seeded, and diced into 1/4-inch (6 mm) cubes

1 yellow bell pepper, cored, seeded, and diced

2 tablespoons (30 ml) lime juice

15 cilantro leaves

PAPAYA CONTAINS PAPAIN, AN ENZYME THAT BREAKS DOWN PROTEINS. PAPAIN IS SO EFFECTIVE THAT POWDERED FORMS OF THE ENZYME ARE USED IN COMMERCIAL MEAT TENDERIZER PRODUCTS. WHEN EATEN AS PART OF A MIXED MEAL, SUCH AS WITH PROTEIN-CONTAINING FOODS SUCH AS CHICKEN, PAPAIN-RICH PAPAYA CAN HELP FACILITATE THE STOMACH'S NATURAL DIGESTIVE PROCESSES. ALL THAT AND IT TASTES GOOD, TOO!

TO PREPARE THE MARINADE: Combine all of the marinade ingredients except the oregano in a large pot. Heat over medium heat until it barely simmers, and then remove from the heat. Allow to cool completely, and then add the oregano.

TO MAKE THE CHICKEN: Place the chicken breasts in a plastic container and cover with the marinade. Refrigerate, covered, overnight. Any extra marinade can be refrigerated and saved in an airtight container for up to a week.

When ready to cook, remove the chicken breasts from the marinade and place them on a sheet pan lined with plastic wrap or parchment paper. Discard the marinade and let the chicken come to room temperature before grilling.

Preheat your grill to medium heat. Once the grill is ready, place the breasts on the grill, skin side down, over direct heat. Let the chicken cook for 5 minutes with the grill lid open. Turn the chicken breasts 90 degrees and cook for an additional 5 minutes. Flip the chicken over and move them to indirect heat. Cook for 10 more minutes, or until the internal temperature of the meat is 165ºF (74ºC). Remove the chicken from the grill and let the meat rest, covered, for 8 minutes.

TO MAKE THE AVOCADO AND PAPAYA SALAD: Combine the avocado, papaya, yellow pepper, lime juice, and cilantro in a mixing bowl and stir. When ready to serve, slice each chicken breast into 4 pieces and top with the salad.

YIELD: 4 SERVINGS

SLIMPALATE'S SIGNATURE SUGAR-FREE BARBECUE SAUCE:

2 tablespoons (32 g) tomato paste

¹/₂ teaspoon ground cinnamon

¹/₄ teaspoon cayenne pepper

¹/₂ medium onion, diced

3 cloves garlic, minced

¹/₄ cup (60 ml) apple cider vinegar

1 teaspoon mustard powder

1 teaspoon cumin

1 teaspoon red chile powder

³/₄ teaspoon smoked paprika

2 tablespoons (30 ml) macadamia nut oil

Salt and pepper to taste

Chicken broth or stock, as needed

FOR CHICKEN:

3-pound (1.4 kg) whole chicken, spatchcocked (see Note)

BUTTERFLIED "SPATCHCOCK" STYLE, THIS CHICKEN WILL COOK UP QUICKLY WITH CRISPY SKIN AND SUPER JUICY MEAT. TO MAKE IT EVEN BETTER, IT'S BASTED WITH SLIMPALATE.COM'S SIGNATURE SUGAR-FREE BARBECUE SAUCE.

Preheat one side of a grill to high heat. If using coals, move all coals to one side of the grill. Put a cast-iron skillet on the grill grate and close the lid.

TO MAKE THE SAUCE: Combine all the sauce ingredients in a blender, blending until very smooth. If needed, use chicken broth to thin the sauce. Coat the entire chicken with the sauce, reserving the rest.

TO MAKE THE CHICKEN: Once the grill is hot, place the chicken, skin side down, over direct heat, weighting it down with the cast-iron skillet (don't forget to use your grilling mitts to move the skillet!). Cook for 6 to 10 minutes. Flip the chicken, weight it down with the skillet again, and grill for another 8 to 10 minutes. Remove the skillet and baste the entire chicken with the sauce.

Place the chicken, skin side down, on the opposite side of the grill and cook for an additional 15 to 20 minutes over indirect heat.

When the chicken is done, transfer to a platter and allow to rest for 5 minutes before carving.

YIELD: 4 TO 6 SERVINGS

"You could probably get through life without knowing how to roast a chicken, but the question is, would you want to?"
–NIGELLA LAWSON

WHAT THE HECK IS A SPATCHCOCKED CHICKEN?

A spatchcocked chicken is simply a butterflied whole chicken. You can ask your butcher to do this for you, or you can do it yourself by removing the backbone with cooking shears, opening the chicken up, and pressing it flat.

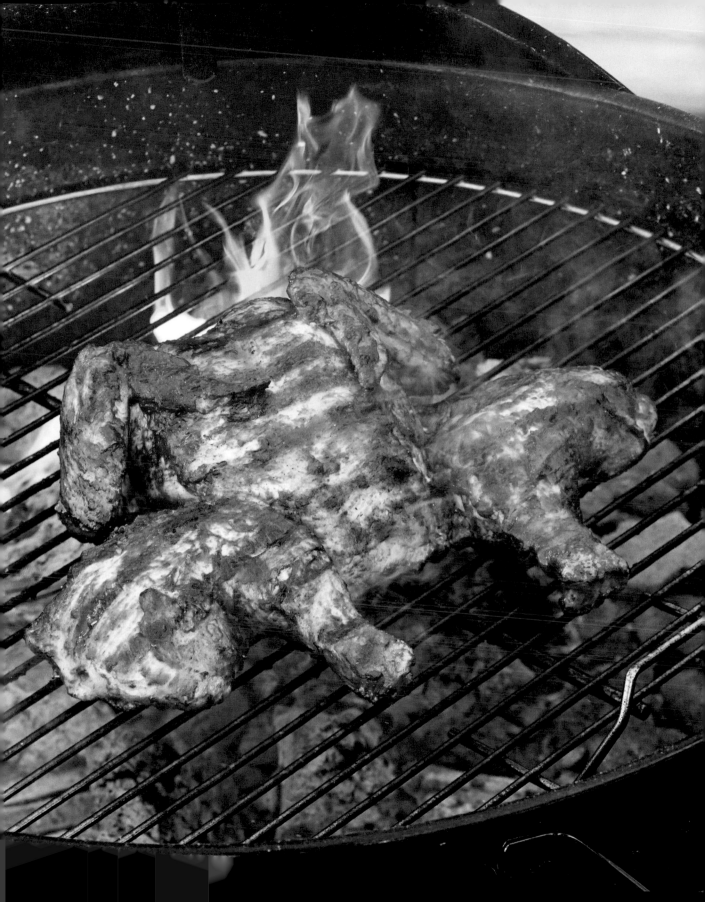

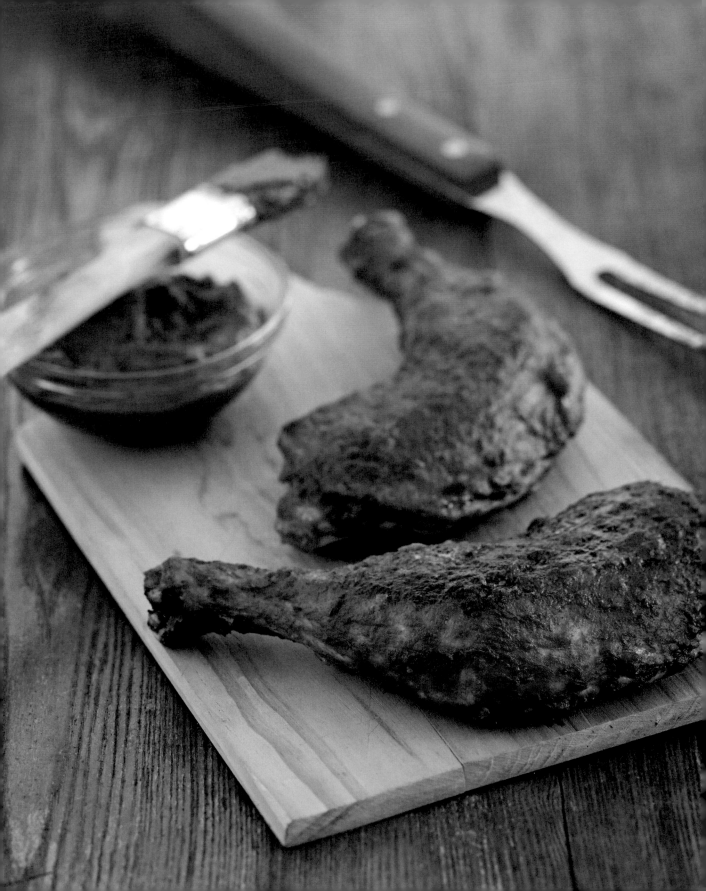

TEXAS OAK BARBECUED CHICKEN LEGS

6 whole chicken legs (about 2¹/₂ pounds [1.1 kg])

2 tablespoons (28 g) lard

4 tablespoons (28 g) Poultry Rub (page 49)

1 cup (240 g) Caveman 'Cue (page 45)

¼ pound (113 g) oak chunks (preferred) or chips

Aluminum pan and hot water (optional)

Aluminum foil (if using wood chips without a smoker box)

ALTHOUGH MESQUITE WOOD IS A TEXAS TRADITION, THE HEAVY SWEET SMOKE CAN SOMETIMES OVERPOWER MILDER MEATS. OAK, ON THE OTHER HAND, HAS A MILDER FLAVOR THAT GOES WELL WITH POULTRY.

Rub the chicken legs with lard and coat with a generous amount of rub.

Prepare your grill for smoking (see "Smoking Without a Smoker" on page 31) and place the chicken legs, skin side down, over direct heat. Allow the chicken legs to cook for 5 minutes and then turn them 90 degrees. Cook for another 5 minutes before flipping the chicken legs and moving them to the top rack of the grill (or the indirect heat side if you don't have a top rack). Brush the chicken liberally with sauce and add about 2 ounces (56 g) of wood chunks/chips on top of the hot coals. For a gas grill, you can simply add the wood chips to your smoker box and place directly over a burner on one side. Close the grill lid.

As the meat cooks, adjust the intake damper vents to keep the temperature of the grill around the meat as close to 225°F (107°C) as you can. You may need to also add more coals to keep the temperature up. Add about 6 hot coals and 2 ounces (56 g) of wood every 30 minutes or so to maintain the temperature. (Note: This is a good time to baste the legs with sauce.) Cracking the lid of the grill, or adding an additional pan full of water to the top grate, can also help if the temperature is running too hot.

Cooking time should run about 90 minutes per pound (450 g), or about 4 hours, and the meat is done when it reaches an internal temperature of 165°F (73°C) and the juices run clear.

Before serving, brush once more with the sauce.

YIELD: 6 SERVINGS

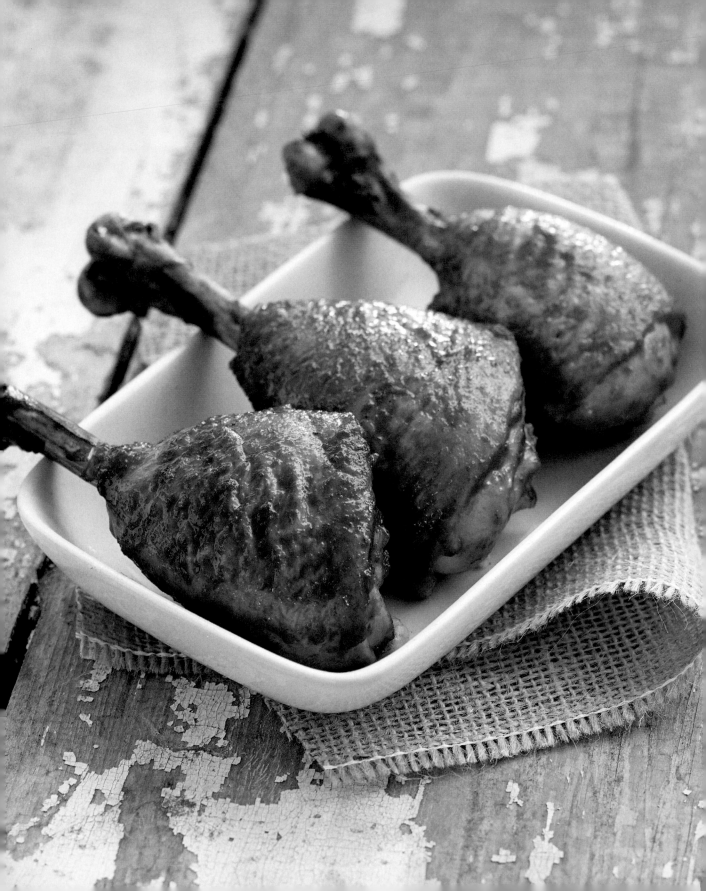

SMOKED CHICKEN LOLLIPOPS

20 chicken "drumettes"

1 cup (108 g) Poultry Rub (page 49)

¼ pound (113 g) applewood chunks

Large aluminum pan and hot water (optional)

Aluminum foil (if using wood chips without a smoker box)

Spray bottle filled with half apple juice, half water

1 cup (240 g) Caveman 'Cue (page 45)

EATING BBQ CHICKEN LEGS TYPICALLY MEANS LOTS OF MESS AND LOTS OF PAPER TOWELS. TURNING THEM INTO EASILY HANDLED "LOLLIPOPS" TAKES CARE OF THIS PROBLEM BY MAKING THEM EASY TO EAT. SMOKING THESE MEATY LOLLIPOPS ALSO MAKES THEM INCREDIBLY FLAVORFUL.

Coat the drumettes with the rub, then, using a sharp knife, cut the skin and tendons around the knuckle of each drumette in a circular motion. Make sure you have cut all of the way to the bone. Push the meat down to the fat end and press the drumette against the cutting board firmly so that it stands with the bone pointed up. Place the "lollipops" in a disposable aluminum pan and refrigerate, covered, for 6 to 12 hours.

When ready to cook, remove the pan of chicken from the refrigerator and allow to return to roo temperature.

Prepare your grill for smoking (see "Smoking Without a Smoker" on page 31) and add about 2 ounces (56 g) of wood chunks on top of the hot coals. For a gas grill, you can simply add the wood chips to your smoker box and place directly over a burner on one side.

Punch a few holes in the bottom of the aluminum pan holding the chicken and place it on the side of the grill receiving indirect heat (over the water pan if you are using one) and close the lid of the grill. As the meat cooks, adjust the intake damper vents to keep the temperature of the grill around the meat as close to 225°F (107°C) as you can. You may need to also add more coals to keep the temperature up. Add about 6 hot coals and 2 ounces (56 g) of wood every 30 minutes or so to maintain the temperature. Cracking the lid of the grill, or adding an additional pan full of water to the top grate, can also help if the temperature is running too hot. Cooking time should run about 90 minutes per pound (450 g) and the meat is done when it reaches an internal temperature of 165°F (73°C), the juices run clear, and the meat pulls easily off the bone.

When ready to serve, place the chicken lollipops on a platter with a ramekin of the barbecue sauce.

YIELD: 5 TO 10 SERVINGS

CRISPY SKIN CHICKEN BREAST

1 herb mop (4 ounces [112 g] fresh thyme sprigs, 4 ounces [112 g] fresh sage leaves, and 4 ounces [112 g] fresh rosemary sprigs bound at one end with butcher's twine)

1 cup (235 ml) olive oil

4 chicken breasts, skin on

Freshly ground black pepper

1 lemon, cut in half

2 tablespoons (5 g) chopped fresh thyme

GRILLING DOESN'T ALWAYS HAVE TO INVOLVE CHARRING, HEAVY RUBS, AND SPICY SAUCES. IN THIS RECIPE, A SUBTLE, UNDERSTATED FLAVOR IS CREATED BY USING AN HERB "MOP" MADE FROM FRESH HERBS DIPPED IN OLIVE OIL. THIS WILL GIVE THE MEAT A HINT OF HERB FLAVOR AND AROMA THAT ENHANCES ITS NATURAL TASTE WITHOUT OVERWHELMING IT.

Preheat the grill to high heat. While waiting, let the ends of the herb mop sit in the olive oil.

When the grill is ready, season the chicken breasts with black pepper and brush lightly with the herb mop. Place the breasts, skin side down, over direct heat for 2 minutes. Turn the chicken breasts 90 degrees and baste again with the olive oil from the herb mop. Allow the chicken breasts to cook for 2 more minutes before flipping and moving to indirect heat. Baste the chicken again and cook for another 8 to 10 minutes, or until the internal temperature reaches 165ºF (74ºC) or the juices run clear when the meat is pierced. Remove the chicken breasts from the grill and allow to rest for 5 minutes.

Before serving, squeeze lemon juice over each piece and sprinkle with fresh thyme.

YIELD: 4 SERVINGS

PULLED CHICKEN STUFFED PEPPERS

1 pound (454 g) chicken from Dijon Chicken with Arugula and Cherry Tomatoes (page 124)

1/2 cup (120 g) Caveman 'Cue Sauce (page 45)

4 bell peppers, any color

1 tablespoon (15 ml) olive oil

BELL PEPPERS ARE LOADED WITH NUTRIENTS MAKE CONVENIENT AND EDIBLE CONTAINERS FOR OTHER FOODS.

Prepare the grilled chicken as described in Dijon Chicken with Arugula and Cherry Tomatoes (page 124). When cool enough to handle, remove 1 pound (454 g) of meat and put it in a large mixing bowl. Add the sauce and mix thoroughly, pulling the meat apart into strands.

Using a sharp knife, cut the peppers in half lengthwise and remove the core, stem, and white pith from the inside of each pepper. Overstuff one side of the pepper with the chicken mixture and cover with the remaining half of the pepper. Tie the pepper together using baker's twine. Repeat with the remaining peppers.

Preheat the grill to medium heat. Rub the peppers lightly with the olive oil and grill for 15 to 20 minutes. Remove from the heat and, using scissors or kitchen shears, cut away the twine. Serve with a knife and fork.

YIELD: 4 SERVINGS

BLACKENED CHICKEN BREASTS

1 1/2 tablespoons (11 g) smoked paprika

1 tablespoon (9 g) granulated garlic

1 tablespoon (7 g) dehydrated onion

1 tablespoon (4.3 g) ground thyme

1 teaspoon freshly ground black pepper

1 teaspoon ground chipotle chile pepper

1/2 teaspoon sea salt

4 boneless, skinless chicken breasts

1/4 cup (60 ml) olive oil

2 lemons, cut in half

BLACKENING ADDS AN INCREDIBLE FLAVOR AND TEXTURE TO MEAT, BUT IT CAN EASILY GO WRONG. TO KEEP FROM BLACKENING YOUR HANDS AND FOREARMS, USE LONG TONGS AND GLOVES!

Preheat the grill to high and put a cast-iron skillet directly over the coals or gas flame. Allow the skillet to heat up for 30 minutes.

In a small bowl, combine the paprika, garlic, onion, thyme, black pepper, chile pepper, and salt. Rub the chicken breasts with the olive oil and then coat on all sides with the seasoning mix.

Carefully place the chicken breasts in the skillet. Pour a small amount of olive oil over each piece and let the chicken cook for 2 minutes, then flip them over. Using grill mitts, move the skillet to indirect heat and allow the chicken to continue cooking until the internal temperature reaches 165°F (74°C) or the juices run clear when the meat is pierced. Before serving, squeeze fresh lemon over each piece.

YIELD: 4 SERVINGS

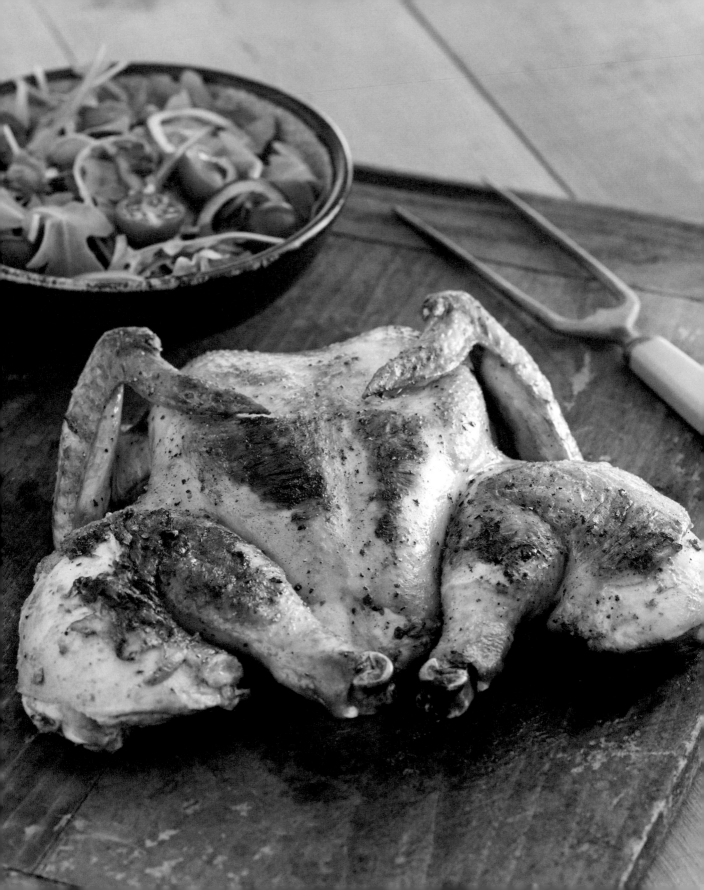

DIJON CHICKEN
WITH ARUGULA AND CHERRY TOMATOES

8 slices bacon, ¹/₄ inch
(6 mm) thick

1 whole chicken

3 tablespoons (33 g)
Dijon mustard

8 sprigs thyme, leaves
picked and chopped

1 teaspoon finely ground
black pepper

6 ounces (170 g) arugula,
rinsed and dried

3 tablespoons (45 ml) extra
virgin olive oil

1 pint (300 g) cherry tomatoes,
cut in half

¹/₂ red onion, thinly sliced

THIS CHICKEN DISH BRINGS LOADS OF FLAVOR, WITH BRIGHT PEPPERY GREENS, FRUITY TOMATOES, AND SALTY BACON.

Cut the bacon into pieces ¹/₂ inch (1.3 cm) wide. Render the bacon in a skillet over medium heat until crispy. Drain the bacon and reserve the fat.

Remove the backbone of the chicken by cutting on each side of it through the cavity using a stiff boning knife, meat shears, or chef's knife. Cut along the cartilage between the breasts and remove. Discard the backbone and cartilage and lay the chicken open. Using a brush, apply the mustard to the inside of the chicken, but not the skin. Sprinkle the chopped thyme and pepper evenly over the mustard.

Preheat the grill to high heat and place the chicken, skinside down, over direct heat. Cook for 2 minutes, turn 90 degrees, and cook for 2 minutes longer. Flip the chicken, season with black pepper, and repeat. Move the chicken to indirect heat and baste with the reserved bacon fat, making sure that the dripping fat doesn't cause flare-ups. Place the lid on the grill, only lifting it to baste every 5 minutes.

After 20 minutes, remove the chicken from the grill and place on a cutting board. If the juices run clear, the chicken is done. Cut the chicken into quarters while still hot and top with the arugula, extra virgin olive oil, cherry tomatoes, red onion, and bacon.

YIELD: 2 TO 4 SERVINGS

MARTHA'S MIX CHICKEN THIGHS

FOR CHICKEN:

8 chicken thighs

1 tablespoon (15 ml) olive oil

1/2 cup (100 g) Martha's Mix Spice Blend (or substitute Citrus and Herb Seafood Rub on page 49, but use lime zest instead of the lemon called for in the rub)

FOR HERB MOP:

4 ounces (112 g) fresh thyme sprigs

4 ounces (112 g) fresh sage leaves

4 ounces (112 g) fresh rosemary sprigs

1/4 cup (60 ml) olive oil

MARTHA'S MIX IS A SPICE BLEND THAT WAS FORMULATED BY SCOTT AND NIKKI KIMBLETON. YOU CAN PURCHASE MARTHA'S MIX DIRECTLY FROM THEIR WEBSITE AT WWW.MARTHASMIX.COM.

TO MAKE THE CHICKEN: Rub the chicken thighs with the olive oil and season generously with Martha's Mix. Place them in a freezer bag and allow them to marinate in the refrigerator overnight.

When ready to cook, preheat your grill to medium heat.

TO MAKE THE HERB MOP: Tie the herbs together on one end with butcher's twine to form an herb "mop." Dip the herb mop into the olive oil and brush the thighs before placing them on the grill, skin side down. Close the lid and cook for 6 minutes. Flip the thighs and brush again with the herb mop dipped in oil. Repeat this process once more before checking the thighs for doneness. When fully cooked, the internal temperature of the meat closest to the bone will be 165ºF (74ºC) and the juices will run clear.

YIELD: 4 TO 8 SERVINGS

GEORGIA PEACH TURKEY BURGER

2 tablespoons (30 ml) olive oil

2 shallots, minced

1 stalk celery, diced small

1 medium slightly under-ripe peach, pitted and diced small

2 sprigs tarragon, finely chopped

1/2 teaspoon white pepper

1 pound (454 g) ground turkey breast

4 tablespoons (60 g) Paleo Mayo (page 47)

4 large leaves green or red leaf lettuce, washed and dried with a paper towel

PEACH ADDS MOISTURE AND FLAVOR TO THE GROUND TURKEY, A SURPRISING COMBINATION THAT MIGHT BECOME A NEW FAVORITE.

Heat the olive oil in a medium sauté pan over medium-high heat. Add the shallots and celery and sweat for 30 seconds. Next, add the peaches and sauté for 1 minute. The peaches should start to brown a little but still be firm. Take the pan off the heat and stir in the tarragon and white pepper. Transfer the mixture to a small bowl and put it into the refrigerator to cool. When the peach mixture has completely cooled, work it into the ground turkey and form into 4 patties.

Preheat the grill to medium-high heat. Cook the burgers for 5 minutes, flip, and cook another 5 to 8 minutes with the grill lid closed. When done, the internal temperature should be 165ºF (74ºC).

To serve, top each burger with 1 tablespoon (15 g) of Paleo Mayo and wrap with a piece of lettuce, using a toothpick or skewer to secure.

YIELD: 4 SERVINGS

WHOLE ROASTED TURKEY BREAST

1 cup (145 g) toasted pecans, crushed

1 cup (32 g) chopped fresh sage

1 tablespoon (7 g) black pepper

3 tablespoons (45 ml) olive oil

Zest of 3 lemons

8-pound (3.6 kg) turkey breast

TREATING EACH PIECE OF THE TURKEY SEPARATELY, RATHER THAN ROASTING THE ENTIRE BIRD, WILL ALLOW YOU TO MAXIMIZE THE POTENTIAL OF EACH PIECE OF MEAT. THE BREAST, A LEANER CUT, NEEDS SPECIAL ATTENTION IN ORDER TO COME OUT JUICY AND FLAVORFUL RATHER THAN DRY.

Preheat the grill to 300ºF (150ºC). In a small bowl, combine the pecans, sage, black pepper, olive oil, and lemon zest to make a paste. Using gloves, spread the paste over the skin and flesh of the turkey breast. Lay out a large piece of cheesecloth and fold it in half so that the folded end is away from you. Place the turkey breast in the middle of the cheesecloth with the fat end of the breast facing toward the left. Fold the side of the cheesecloth closest to you over the top of the breast and roll the entire turkey breast over the other half. Tie the open ends of the cheesecloth with butcher's twine and make sure the turkey is tightly secured.

Place your turkey breast on the top rack of the grill and close the lid. Cook for 3 to 4 hours, or until the internal temperature is 165ºF (74ºC). Remove from the grill and let rest for 15 minutes on a cutting board. When ready to serve, remove the cheesecloth and cut the turkey breast into thick slices.

YIELD: 20 TO 24 SERVINGS

SMOKED TURKEY LEGS

4 turkey legs

1 gallon (3.6 L) Sweet and Savory Spice Brine (page 53)

¼ pound (113 g) applewood chunks (preferred) or chips

Aluminum pan and hot water (optional)

Aluminum foil (if using wood chips without a smoker box)

IT'S HARD NOT TO FEEL A LITTLE BIT LIKE GROK WHEN YOU'RE WALKING AROUND GNAWING ON A GIANT TURKEY LEG. EATING FOOD WITH YOUR HANDS, GETTING MEAT STUCK IN YOUR TEETH, AND CHEWING ON ALL THE STRINGY BITS IS ONE WAY TO RECONNECT WITH THE PRIMAL EXPERIENCE OF BEING HUMAN AND BEING ALIVE.

Place each turkey leg in a large 1-gallon (3.6 L) freezer bag. Pour 1 quart (940 ml) of the brine into each bag, seal the bags, and refrigerate overnight.

Remove the turkey legs from the freezer bags and discard the brine. Put the turkey legs on a platter and allow them to come to room temperature.

Prepare your grill for smoking (see "Smoking Without a Smoker" on page 31) and add about 2 ounces (56 g) of wood chunks on top of the hot coals. For a gas grill, you can simply add the wood chips to your smoker box and place directly over a burner on one side.

Put the meat on the side of the grill receiving indirect heat (over the water pan if you are using one) and close the lid of the grill. As the meat cooks, adjust the intake damper vents to keep the temperature of the grill around the meat as close to 225°F (107°C) as you can. You may need to also add more coals to keep the temperature up. Add about 6 hot coals and 2 ounces (56 g) of wood every 30 minutes or so to maintain the temperature. Cracking the lid of the grill, or adding an additional pan full of water to the top grate, can also help if the temperature is running too hot. Cooking time should run about 90 minutes per pound (450 g) and the meat is done when it reaches an internal temperature of 165°F (73°C). When finished, the turkey legs should be very dark brown.

Before serving, wrap the turkey legs in foil and let them rest for 10–15 minutes.

YIELD: 4 TO 8 SERVINGS

GRILLED DUCK BREAST WITH SAUERKRAUT

6 duck breasts, skin scored

1 teaspoon ground coriander

1 teaspoon black pepper

1 teaspoon sea salt

1 quart (940 ml) sauerkraut (look for a naturally fermented brand such as Bubbies)

WHEN JAY PHELAN WAS LIVING IN NEW YORK AS A STRUGGLING CULINARY STUDENT, HE HAD TO LEARN HOW TO BE THRIFTY. HE SPENT A LOT OF TIME AT FARMERS' MARKETS AND ON ONE OCCASION CAME ACROSS 10-POUND (4.6 KG) HEADS OF GREEN CABBAGE THAT WERE BEING SOLD FOR A DOLLAR EACH. HE BOUGHT THREE AND LUGGED THEM BACK TO THE APARTMENT HE SHARED WITH SEVEN OTHER CULINARY STUDENTS. AFTER SLICING THEM UP AND JAMMING THEM INTO CONTAINERS FULL OF SALT AND SOME JUNIPER BERRIES, HE PUT THEM UNDER THE SINK, WHERE THEY REMAINED FORGOTTEN UNTIL FOUR WEEKS LATER. WHEN THEY WERE FINALLY REDISCOVERED, HE WAS PLEASANTLY SURPRISED TO FIND FINISHED SAUERKRAUT!

IN ADDITION TO BEING TASTY, NATURALLY FERMENTED SAUERKRAUT IS FULL OF PROBIOTIC BACTERIA AND IS GOOD FOR THE DIGESTIVE SYSTEM. IN THIS DISH, THE TANGY FERMENTED CABBAGE CUTS THE RICHNESS OF THE DUCK BREAST, MAKING THE TWO PERFECT COMPANIONS.

Season the duck breasts with the coriander, pepper, and salt.

Preheat the grill to medium heat. Place the breasts skin side down over direct heat. The flame will flare once the fat starts to render and drip. Be prepared to move the duck breasts immediately to another part of the grill once this happens.

When the skin has taken on a golden brown color, about 5 minutes, move the duck breasts to indirect heat. Cook for 5 more minutes before flipping. Bring the duck back over direct heat for 1 more minute before removing from the grill. When finished, the meat will be rare to medium-rare. Let the duck rest for 5 minutes before slicing against the grain with a sharp knife. Serve over sauerkraut.

YIELD: 6 SERVINGS

"To begin cooking duck at one in the morning is one of the finest acts of madness that can be undertaken by a human being who is not mad."
—MANUEL VÁZQUEZ MONTALBÁN

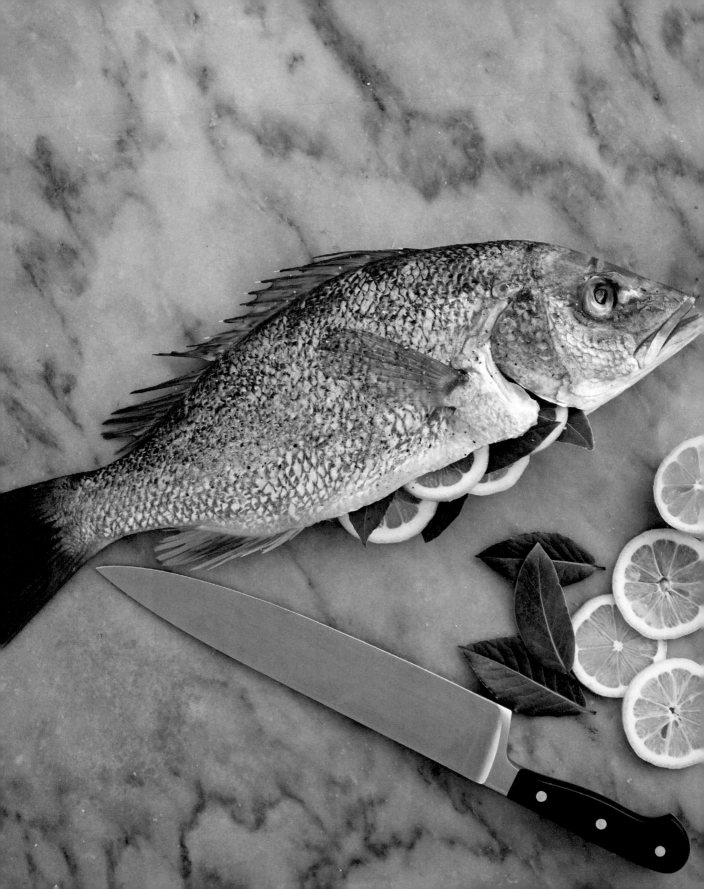

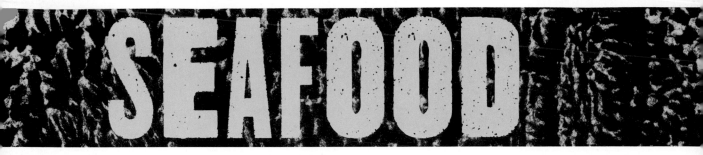

SEAFOOD

**1 pound (454 g) alder
or cedar wood**

**2 whole snapper (1 to 1¹/₂
pounds [454 to 680 g] each),
cleaned, gutted, and scaled**

8 fresh bay leaves

**1 tablespoon (15 ml)
light olive oil**

1 lemon, cut in half

Sea salt

Cracked pink peppercorns

WHOLE SNAPPER
WITH GRILLED LEMON AND BAY LEAF

COOKING FISH ON THE BONE IMPARTS A FLAVOR AND STRUCTURE THAT IS LOST WHEN THE BONES ARE REMOVED PRIOR TO COOKING. BECAUSE OF ITS SIZE AND ABILITY TO TAKE ON WOOD SMOKE, SNAPPER IS OFTEN USED FOR THIS SORT OF RUSTIC APPLICATION. ARCTIC CHAR OR TROUT CAN BE SUBSTITUTED FOR SNAPPER.

This is best done over a wood and charcoal grill. Alder or cedar is the best choice. Preheat the grill to 450°F (232°C).

Rinse the snappers thoroughly and pat dry with paper towels. With a sharp fish knife, cut 3 diagonal slits along both sides of the fish. The cuts should go almost all the way through the flesh. Then, use your knife and carefully loosen the skin from the flesh just enough to be able to insert the bay leaves. Push the bay leaves between the skin and flesh of each fish. Oil the whole fish lightly with olive oil. Place the fish on the grill over indirect heat. Immediately close the lid and allow to cook for 6 to 7 minutes.

Using a flat grill spatula, carefully turn the fish over. Try to do this gently so that the skin on the fish stays intact. At this point, place the lemon halves on the grill over direct heat, flat side down. Close the lid and grill the fish for another 6 to 7 minutes. Transfer the fish and lemon halves to a cutting board. Allow to cool for a couple of minutes. With an 8-inch (20 cm) chef's knife, cut the fish along the spine, following the rib bones to remove the fillet from the fish. Turn it over and do the same on the other side. Repeat with the second fish. Transfer the fillets to a platter and season with sea salt and pink peppercorns. Squeeze the grilled lemon halves over all and serve.

YIELD: 4 SERVINGS

AHI TUNA WITH MACADAMIA PEACH CHUTNEY

FOR MACADAMIA PEACH CHUTNEY:

1 cup (235 ml) apple cider vinegar

2 tablespoons (24 g) coconut sugar

2 peaches, pitted and diced

10 toasted macadamia nuts, crushed

FOR TUNA:

Four 6-ounce (170 g) ahi tuna from the center of the loin, 2 inches (5 cm) thick

Cracked black pepper

Macadamia nut oil, for drizzling

1 avocado, cut in half with pit removed

HIGH-QUALITY, FRESH TUNA IS INCREDIBLE, WHICH IS WHY IT IS OFTEN SERVED RAW AS POKE, TARTARE, OR SASHIMI. HOWEVER, SOMETHING MAGICAL HAPPENS WHEN IT IS SEARED OR GRILLED AT A HIGH TEMPERATURE. NATURALLY OCCURRING SUGARS IN THE FLESH REACT WITH AMINO ACIDS AND FORM HUNDREDS OF DIFFERENT FLAVOR COMPOUNDS.

TO MAKE THE CHUTNEY: Simmer the apple cider vinegar and coconut sugar in a saucepot over medium heat until reduced by half. This should take about 2 minutes. Add the diced peaches and macadamia nuts and simmer for another 2 minutes. Remove the pan from the heat and let it come to room temperature.

TO MAKE THE TUNA: Preheat the grill to medium-high heat. Rub the tuna with the cracked black pepper and drizzle with the macadamia nut oil. Place the tuna over direct heat and sear for 1 minute. Turn the fish 90 degrees and cook for another minute before flipping. Repeat the process on the other side. When done, the tuna should be red and still cool in the center. Transfer the tuna to a cutting board and slice using a very sharp knife.

To serve, arrange slices of tuna on a plate with a spoonful of the chutney. Slice thin pieces of avocado and fan over the tuna.

YIELD: 4 SERVINGS

GRILLED TUNA BELLY

2¹/₂ pounds (1.1 kg) tuna belly

Olive oil, for drizzling

¹/₂ cup (100 g) Citrus and Herb Seafood Rub (page 49)

2 lemons, sliced

TUNA BELLY, ALSO CALLED FATTY TUNA OR TORO, IS VERY RICH AND USED TO BE DISCARDED BY JAPANESE CHEFS WHOSE CUSTOMERS WEREN'T ACCUSTOMED TO EATING OILY CUTS OF THE FISH. RECENTLY, HOWEVER, THE FATTY TUNA BELLY HAS BECOME A PRIZED INGREDIENT, ESPECIALLY WHEN PREPARED AS *ABURI TORO*, LITERALLY "LIGHTLY GRILLED TUNA BELLY." QUICK GRILLING MAKES THE FATTY FISH EVEN CREAMIER AND INTENSIFIES THE FLAVOR.

With a sharp knife, remove the skin from the outer side and some of the thicker pieces of white tissue from the inner side of the tuna belly. Drizzle the tuna with olive oil and season generously with the rub.

Preheat the grill to medium-high heat. Place the tuna belly on a grill rack. If using charcoal, carefully use tongs to place the tuna belly and rack directly onto the coals. If using gas, place the rack over direct heat. Cook the tuna belly for 2 minutes on one side before flipping. Cook for an additional minute and then remove the tuna from the grill. When done, the tuna belly should be somewhat charred on the outside and rare in the middle.

To serve, cut the tuna into 6 pieces and garnish with fresh lemon slices.

YIELD: 6 SERVINGS

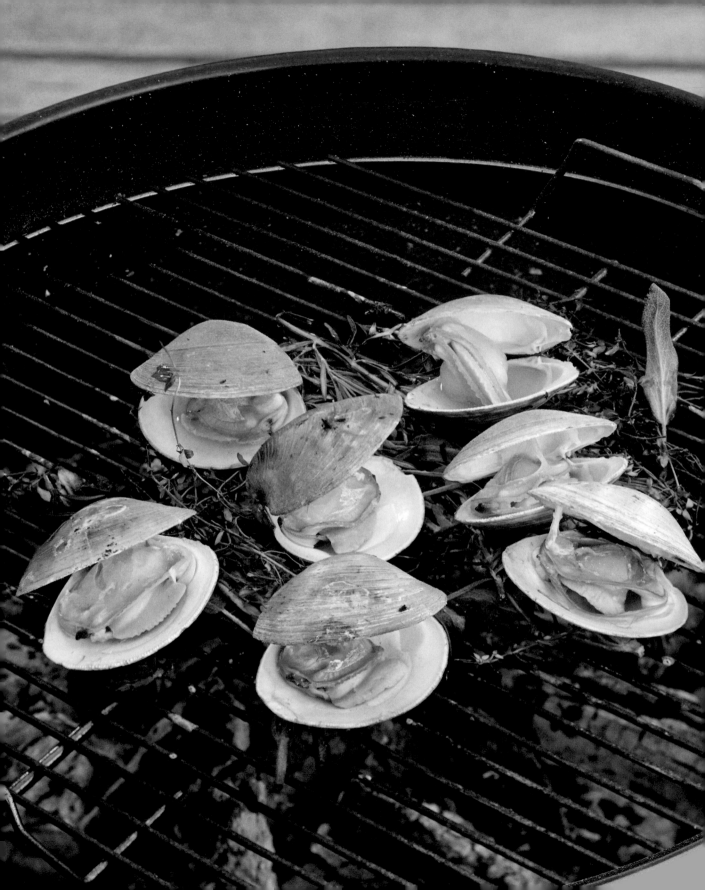

HERB-SMOKED CLAMS

20 sprigs fresh rosemary

8 ounces (227 g) fresh thyme

8 ounces (227 g) fresh sage

1 gallon (3.6 L) water

20 to 24 cherrystone clams (also known as Pacific littleneck, manila, butter, or steamer clams)

8 ounces (227 g) sea salt

Garlic Espelette Aioli (page 75), for serving

Charred Tomatillo Salsa (page 47), for serving

CLAMS ARE SOMETIMES SMOKED WITH PINE BOUGHS, BUT THE THICK PINE RESIN GIVES OFF A STRONG SMOKE THAT CAN BE OVERLY PUNGENT. USING HERBS, HOWEVER, IMPARTS A SUBTLER FLAVOR THAT ALLOWS THE NATURAL AROMAS OF SHELLFISH, SALT, AND SEA TO STAND OUT AS WELL.

Soak all of the herbs in the water for 1 hour. Meanwhile, place the clams in a large plastic container. Put the container of clams in the sink and pour the salt in with them. Run a continuous stream of water over the clams for 1 hour (this will pull the grit out of the clams). Take the clams out of the water and scrub the outside with a brush.

Preheat the grill to medium heat. Remove the herbs from the water and shake off the excess water. Place the herbs over the direct heat, forming a thick bed. Put the clams on top of the herb bed. When the herbs start to catch fire and smoke, cover the grill with the lid. Let smoke for 10 minutes and check. Take off the ones that have opened and let the rest smoke until they open as well. Serve on a platter with cocktail forks and bowls of the aioli and salsa.

YIELD: 2 TO 4 SERVINGS

"As I ate the oysters with their strong taste of the sea and their faint metallic taste that the cold white wine washed away, leaving only the sea taste and the succulent texture, and as I drank their cold liquid from each shell and washed it down with the crisp taste of the wine, I lost the empty feeling and began to be happy and to make plans."
—**ERNEST HEMINGWAY,** A Moveable Feast

GRILLED SWORDFISH WITH JICAMA MANGO SLAW

FOR MANGO JICAMA SLAW:

4 ounces (112 g) jicama, shredded

1 ripe mango, peeled, pitted, and diced small

1 ripe Roma tomato, seeded and diced small

1 scallion, finely sliced

1 small bunch cilantro, roughly chopped

Juice of 1 lime

2 tablespoons (30 ml) avocado oil

FOR SWORDFISH:

Four 6-ounce (170 g) swordfish loin steaks

2 tablespoons (30 ml) avocado oil

1 teaspoon coarsely ground coriander seed

1 teaspoon coarsely ground black pepper

Sea salt

NORTHERN ATLANTIC SWORDFISH IS A GREAT FISH FOR GRILLING OVER A WOOD FLAME. LIKE A STEAK, IT CAN BE ENJOYED PERFECTLY RARE AND WONDERFUL. WHEN COOLED AND THINLY SLICED, IT IS ALMOST LIKE A BEEF CARPACCIO.

TO PREPARE THE MANGO JICAMA SLAW: Combine the jicama, mango, tomato, scallion, cilantro, lime juice, and avocado oil in a bowl. Gently stir until all the ingredients are evenly mixed. Cover the bowl and refrigerate until ready to serve.

TO MAKE THE SWORDFISH: Preheat your grill to high. Rub the swordfish with the avocado oil and season with the coriander, black pepper, and sea salt. Place the steaks on the grill and sear for 2 minutes, turn 90 degrees, and cook for another 2 minutes. Flip and repeat the process on the other side. When done, the swordfish should be medium-rare to medium.

Serve the swordfish while hot and top with the slaw.

YIELD: 4 SERVINGS

BLACK PEPPER WILD SALMON WITH FENNEL APPLE SALAD

FOR FENNEL APPLE SALAD:

1 bulb fennel, thinly sliced, fronds removed

1 Golden Delicious, Empire, or Gala apple, cored and thinly sliced

1 medium orange, peeled and sectioned, white pith completely removed

Juice of 1 lemon

1 tablespoon (15 ml) avocado oil

1 teaspoon snipped chives

FOR SALMON:

4 tablespoons (20 g) black peppercorns, coarsely crushed

Four 6-ounce (170 g) salmon fillets, pin bones removed

2 tablespoons (30 ml) olive oil

THE QUALITY OF COMMERCIALLY AVAILABLE SALMON—INCLUDING FARM RAISED, WILD CAUGHT, ATLANTIC AND PACIFIC SALMON—CAN VARY GREATLY. SOON THERE WILL EVEN BE VARIETIES OF GMO SALMON THAT WILL LIKELY BE UNLABLED DUE TO THE FDA'S UNWILLINGNESS TO SUPPORT CONSUMERS' RIGHT TO CHOOSE WHETHER OR NOT THEY EAT GENETICALLY MODIFIED FOODS. YOUR BEST BET, BOTH FLAVOR AND HEALTHWISE, IS TO CHOOSE WILD-CAUGHT SALMON EVEN THOUGH IT IS MORE EXPENSIVE. IT HAS A RICHER FLAVOR AND A HIGHER CONCENTRATION OF THE ANTIOXIDANT ASTAXANTHIN AS WELL AS OMEGA-3 FATTY ACIDS.

TO MAKE THE FENNEL APPLE SALAD: Combine the fennel, apple, orange sections, lemon juice, avocado oil, and chives in a small bowl. Toss gently and set aside.

TO MAKE THE SALMON: Preheat the grill to medium heat. On a flat plate or sheet pan, evenly spread out the ground peppercorns and push each fillet flesh side down into the pepper. Drizzle the fillets with olive oil and place on the grill, peppercorn side down. Grill over direct heat for 3 minutes before carefully flipping. Grill for another 3 minutes, or until the fish starts to flake when tested with a fork.

To serve, place the fillets on plates with the peppercorn-crusted side facing up and top with portion of the fennel apple salad.

YIELD: 4 SERVINGS

PULPO A LA PARRILLA

FOR OCTOPUS:

2 gallons (7.2 L) water

2 lemons, cut in half

1 bunch flat-leaf parsley, stems and leaves separated, chopped

1 bulb garlic, cut in half

2-pound (908 g) octopus, cleaned of innards and brain

FOR MARINADE:

2 tablespoons (20 g) minced garlic

1 tablespoon (7 g) paprika

1 cup (235 ml) sherry vinegar

1 cup (235 ml) extra virgin olive oil

THE OCTOPUS DOESN'T HAVE A SKELETON, BUT IT IS INCREDIBLY STRONG DUE TO ITS DENSE MUSCLES AND CONNECTIVE TISSUE. THIS GIVES OCTOPUS MEAT A UNIQUE TEXTURE AND DENSITY THAT IS UNLIKE EITHER FISH OR SHELLFISH. IT IS DELICIOUS NONETHELESS, ESPECIALLY WHEN PROPERLY PREPARED!

TO MAKE THE OCTOPUS: In a large pot, combine the water, lemons, parsley stems, and garlic. Bring the water to a boil over high heat and gently lower the octopus into the water, tentacles first. The tentacles will tighten up and curl immediately as they start to cook. When the water returns to a boil, lower the temperature to a simmer and cook for 45 minutes to 1 hour. (Boiling 30 minutes per 1 pound [454 g] is the general rule for octopus.) When the octopus is done simmering, drain in a colander and let cool to room temperature. When cool enough to handle, cut the octopus into large sections.

Preheat your grill to high heat. Place the octopus sections on the grill and cook them over direct heat until they become slightly charred, 2 to 3 minutes. Turn over and slightly char the other side. Remove the octopus from the grill and let it cool.

TO MAKE THE MARINADE: In a medium-size bowl, whisk together the minced garlic, paprika, vinegar, and olive oil. Add the octopus to the marinade, cover the bowl, and refrigerate overnight.

When ready to serve, remove the octopus from the marinade and thinly slice. Place on a serving plate and garnish with the remaining parsley leaves.

YIELD: 8 SERVINGS

UNCLE KEITH'S FLORIDA LOBSTER TAILS

4 Florida lobster tails

$1/2$ teaspoon cayenne pepper

2 teaspoons (12 g) sea salt

Zest of 1 lemon

1 ounce (28 g) minced garlic

$1/4$ cup (60 ml) avocado oil

2 lemons, cut in half

THIS RECIPE COMES FROM KEITH GIBBS, A GOOD FRIEND OF JAY PHELAN. KEITH FLIES HIS PLANE TO THE BAHAMAS A FEW TIMES A YEAR AND SPENDS EQUAL AMOUNTS OF TIME RELAXING AND DIVING FOR FLORIDA LOBSTERS. HIS RECIPE IS AN INCREDIBLE WAY TO COOK FLORIDA LOBSTER TAILS BECAUSE THE LOWER COOKING TEMPERATURE GIVES THE MEAT A VERY BUTTERY TEXTURE.

Preheat a charcoal grill with coals piled up in the center. You should be able to hold your hand 3 inches (7.5 cm) over the grill for about 2 seconds. Using kitchen shears, cut lengthwise along the back of the lobster shells. Flip the tails over and cut along the underside of the tails as well. Use a chef's knife to cut through the tail meat and back fans, leaving the shell around the meat.

Combine the cayenne pepper, sea salt, lemon zest, and garlic in a small bowl and sprinkle over the flesh of each lobster tail. It may not seem like much seasoning, but the lobster doesn't need much. Drizzle the avocado oil over the meat, making sure that it is caught by the shell. Arrange the lobster tails around the outside of the grill, over indirect heat. Close the grill lid and cook for 5 to 6 minutes, or until the meat has just started to pull away from the shell. When the lobsters are done, remove them from the grill and loosen the tail meat from the shell. Serve garnished with fresh lemon.

YIELD: 2 TO 4 SERVINGS

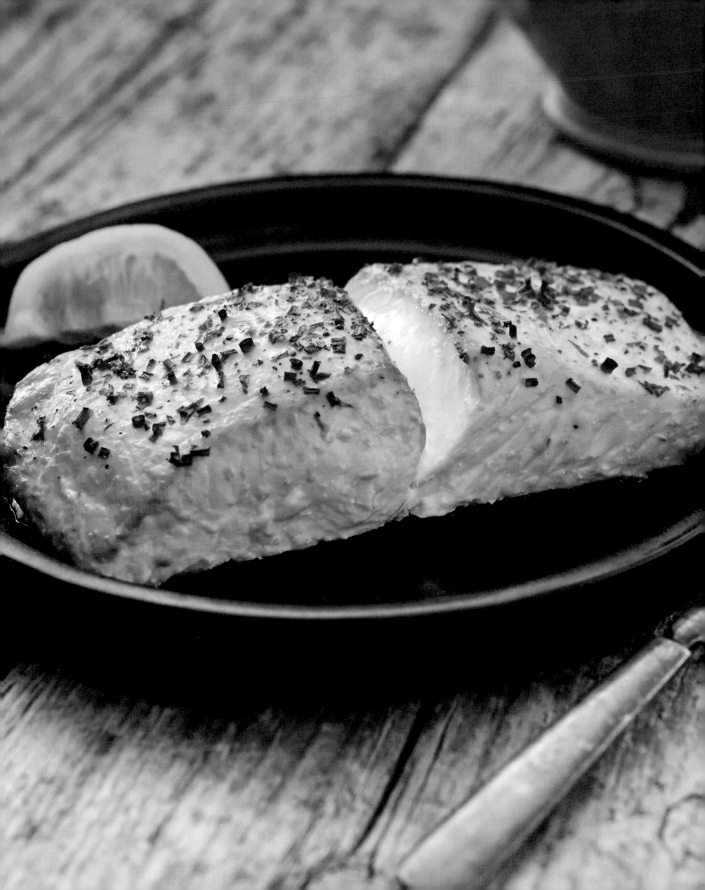

CEDAR PLANK HALIBUT

16 x 18-inch (40 x 45 cm)
cedarwood plank

2-pound (908 g) halibut fillet

Sea salt and black pepper

1 teaspoon minced chives

1 teaspoon minced tarragon

CEDAR PLANKS ARE EASY TO FIND, BUT ALDER, OAK, OR MAPLE WOOD ALSO WORK GREAT FOR THIS DISH. USING CEDAR AND OTHER TYPES OF WOOD TO GRILL HAS ITS ROOTS WITH THE NATIVE AMERICANS OF THE PACIFIC NORTHWEST. OUT OF NECESSITY, THEY WOULD TIE FISH OR GAME TO LARGE PLANKS OF WOOD AND ALLOW THE INDIRECT HEAT OF AN OPEN FIRE TO COOK THE MEAT. THAT THIS TECHNIQUE ALSO FLAVORS FOOD IS A HAPPY ACCIDENT THAT THEY, AND BY EXTENSION WE, CAN BE THANKFUL FOR.

Soak the cedar plank in water to cover for 1 hour. Preheat the grill to medium heat. Remove the plank from the water and pat dry. Place the halibut on the plank and season with sea salt and pepper. Scatter the chives and tarragon evenly over the fillet. Place the plank and halibut directly over the flame. Cover the grill with the lid and cook for 20 minutes, or until the halibut just starts to flake when tested with a fork.

YIELD: 4 SERVINGS

GRILLED OYSTERS

24 medium-size oysters

1 cup (280 g) Charred Tomatillo Salsa (page 47)

APALACHICOLA, FLORIDA, IS A SMALL TOWN IN APALACHICOLA BAY ABOUT 80 MILES (130 KM) SOUTHWEST OF THE STATE CAPITAL TALLAHASSEE. IT SITS WHERE THE APALACHICOLA RIVER DUMPS RICH, SEDIMENT-FILLED WATER INTO A SHALLOW, WARM BAY, MAKING IT THE PERFECT ENVIRONMENT FOR OYSTERS. IF YOU CAN FIND THEM, THEY ARE HIGHLY RECOMMENDED FOR THIS RECIPE.

Prepare your oysters by first checking to see whether any are open. If they are, that means the oyster has already died and should be discarded. Keep the oysters that are still tightly closed and rinse and scrub the outside of the shell with a coarse brush under cold water.

Preheat the grill to high heat. If using charcoal, arrange the coals evenly to create uniform heat across the entire grill. Place the oysters on the grill and close the lid. Check frequently. As soon as the first oyster pops open, remove them all from the heat with tongs, being careful not to spill the juices contained in the shell. Pry open the oysters the rest of the way using an oyster knife or paring knife. Lightly and carefully detach the muscle that connects the oyster to the shell. Leave the meat of the oyster in the half-shell and transfer to a platter.

To serve, top each oyster with a small amount of the salsa.

YIELD: 4 TO 6 SERVINGS

GRILLED SOFT-SHELL CRAB BLT

4 soft-shell crabs, face, back central apron, and gills removed

2 tablespoons (30 ml) olive oil

¼ cup (60 g) Paleo Mayo (page 47)

8 slices bacon, cooked until crispy

10 leaves Bibb lettuce

1 large beefsteak tomato, thinly sliced

Black pepper

THE *B* IN *BLT* DOESN'T STAND FOR "BUN." HERE, IT'S ALL ABOUT THE BACON, LETTUCE, AND TOMATO—SANDWICHED BETWEEN TWO GRILLED SOFT-SHELLED CRABS! YOU'RE PROBABLY GOING TO NEED A KNIFE AND FORK FOR THIS SANDWICH, THOUGH.

Preheat the grill to medium heat with an area for indirect heat. Lightly rub the crabs with the oil and place them on the grill over direct heat, shell side down. When the edges start to slightly char, flip the crabs over and place over indirect heat. Close the grill lid and cook for 5 minutes.

Remove the crabs from the grill and place two of the crabs shell side down. Coat the crabs with the mayo and top each with 4 slices of bacon, 5 lettuce leaves, and 2 slices of tomato. Crack black pepper over the tomato. Coat the underside of the remaining 2 crabs with mayo before using them to top the BLT.

YIELD: 2 SERVINGS

GRILLED WHOLE BABY FLOUNDER WITH COCONUT RED CURRY

Two 1- to 2-pound (454 to 908 g) whole flounder, cleaned and gutted, fins and tail removed

Olive oil

1 cup (235 ml) Coconut Red Curry Sauce (page 53)

THE BOTTOM-FEEDING FLOUNDER ACTUALLY STARTS ITS LIFE LOOKING MUCH LIKE OTHER FISH, WITH EYES POSITIONED ON BOTH SIDES OF ITS HEAD. AS IT MATURES, ONE EYE GRADUALLY MOVES TO ONE SIDE, ALLOWING THE FISH TO LIE FLAT ON THE OCEAN FLOOR. AS STRANGE AS THIS IS, FLOUNDER HAS A DELICIOUS FLESH THAT MAKES IT PERFECT FOR GRILLING. THE COCONUT RED CURRY SAUCE ADDS A LEVEL OF REFINEMENT TO AN OTHERWISE RUSTIC PREPARATION.

Preheat the grill to high heat with an area for indirect heat. Rub the fish with the olive oil and place over direct heat, dark side down. Cook for 3 minutes, turn the fish 90 degrees, and cook for an additional 3 minutes. Flip the fish and repeat the process on the other side. Move the fish to indirect heat and allow it to cook for 5 more minutes, or until the flesh flakes off the bone when tested with a fork. You can test this by pushing a fork into the middle of the fish and pulling it slightly toward you.

Warm the sauce in a small saucepot over low heat. Transfer the fish to a serving platter and pour the warm sauce over the top.

YIELD: 2 TO 4 SERVINGS

GRAPE LEAF–WRAPPED GRILLED TROUT

24 grape leaves

Six 14- to 16-ounce (392 to 454 g) whole trout, cleaned and gutted

Sea salt and coarsely ground black pepper

12 sprigs fresh thyme

4 lemons, thinly sliced, divided

6 tablespoons (90 ml) olive oil

1 pound (454 g) oak wood chips, soaked in water or apple juice

WRAPPING FISH IN GRAPE OR BANANA LEAVES IS AN ANCIENT TECHNIQUE THAT FLAVORS THE FISH AND KEEPS IT MOIST. TROUT IS CALLED FOR IN THIS RECIPE, BUT THIS METHOD CAN BE USED FOR ANY SMALLER FISH THAT TENDS TO BECOME OVERCOOKED AND DRY, SUCH AS ARCTIC CHAR.

Soak 12 wooden skewers in water to cover for 30 minutes (or use metal skewers).

Bring a large pot of water to a boil, add the grape leaves, and blanch for 1 minute. Carefully remove them from the water and place on paper towels to dry.

Season the inside of the fish with sea salt and black pepper and place 2 thyme sprigs and 6 lemon slices inside the cavity of each fish. Wrap each fish with 4 grape leaves and secure with the skewers by running the points diagonally through the belly of the fish. Drizzle the outside of the leaves and exposed pieces of fish with olive oil.

Preheat the grill to medium heat and create a section for both indirect and direct cooking. If using charcoal, add the oak chips directly to the coals; if using gas, put the chips into a smoker box over direct heat.

Grill the fish for 3 to 4 minutes over direct heat, then flip and cook for an additional 3 to 4 minutes. Transfer the fish to the section with indirect heat and close the grill lid. Cook for 15 to 20 minutes, or until the flesh flakes easily when tested with a fork. Remove from the grill and carefully pull out the skewers. Open the grape leaves and remove the thyme and lemon from the inside of the fish.

To serve, rewrap the fish in the grape leaves and place on plates with the remaining fresh lemon slices.

YIELD: 6 SERVINGS

GRILLED BABY SQUID

16 baby squid, each 2 to 3 inches (5 to 7.5 cm) long, cleaned

$^1/_4$ cup (60 ml) olive oil

2 teaspoons (6 g) minced garlic

1 teaspoon paprika

Sea salt

Juice of 1 lemon

1 tablespoon (2 g) finely chopped fresh marjoram or oregano

COOKING SQUID CAN GO VERY RIGHT OR VERY WRONG. LIKE ITS COUSIN THE OCTOPUS, SQUID ARE EXCELLENT IF PROPERLY PREPARED, BUT THEY HAVE A TENDENCY TO TURN TOUGH AND RUBBERY IF OVERCOOKED. FOR THIS RECIPE, YOU'LL NEED TO BE MINDFUL OF FLARE-UPS BECAUSE OF THE OLIVE OIL USED IN THE MARINADE. JUST IN CASE, KEEP A SPRAY BOTTLE OF WATER HANDY TO KEEP THEM UNDER CONTROL.

Put the squid in a medium-size bowl, and in a separate bowl, whisk together the olive oil, garlic, paprika, and salt. Reserve half of the mixture and pour the other half over the squid. Add the lemon juice and marjoram to the reserved half and set aside. Allow the squid to sit in the marinade for 5 minutes.

Preheat the grill to high heat and place a mesh grill screen over the grate. Place the squid on the grill screen one by one. If they start to flare, spray the flame lightly with the water from the spray bottle, being careful not to be overzealous with the water or the squid will steam and lose their grilled flavor. After 2 to 3 minutes, turn the squid over and grill for an additional 2 minutes.

To serve, place the grilled squid on a serving dish and top with the reserved oil and herb mixture.

YIELD: 4 TO 6 SERVINGS

CRAB-STUFFED PIMIENTOS

2 tablespoons (30 g) Paleo Mayo (page 47)

1 teaspoon paprika

1 teaspoon chopped fresh tarragon

Zest of 1 lemon

Pinch of Aleppo or cayenne pepper

1 pound (454 g) lump or jumbo lump crabmeat, cleaned of all shell

8 to 10 pimiento peppers jarred in olive oil

15 leaves fresh arugula

3 tablespoons (45 ml) White Balsamic Vinaigrette (page 52)

PIMIENTO PEPPERS ARE SIMILAR TO BELL PEPPERS AND ARE BEST KNOWN FOR BEING STUFFED INTO OLIVES. IN THIS RECIPE IT'S THE PIMIENTOS THAT ARE GETTING STUFFED WITH SWEET CRABMEAT AND FLAVORFUL SPICES.

In a small bowl, combine the mayo, paprika, tarragon, and lemon zest until smooth and homogeneous and season with pinch of hot pepper. Gently fold in the crab, being careful not to break up the meat. Remove the pimientos from the jar and spoon the crab mixture into them, leaving a little room at the opening.

Preheat the grill to high heat. Place a wire mesh or grill screen over the grill grate. Place the stuffed pimientos over direct heat and cook for 2 minutes before carefully flipping. Grill the pimientos for 1 minute longer before removing from the heat. When done, the crab stuffing should be warm but not hot.

To serve, lightly dress the arugula with the vinaigrette. Put a portion of the dressed arugula onto each plate and top with 2 pimientos.

YIELD: 4 OR 5 SERVINGS

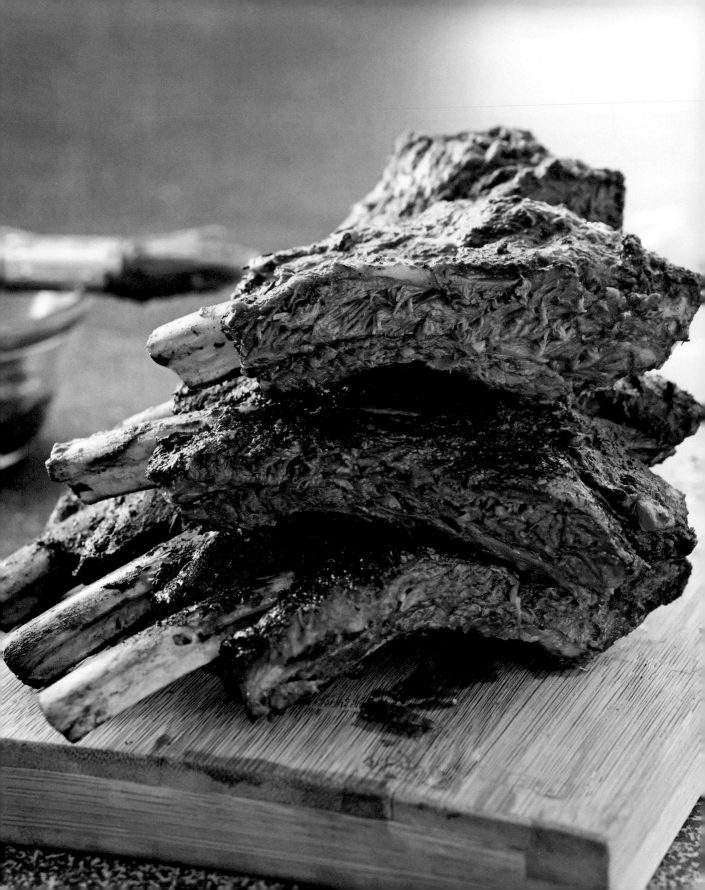

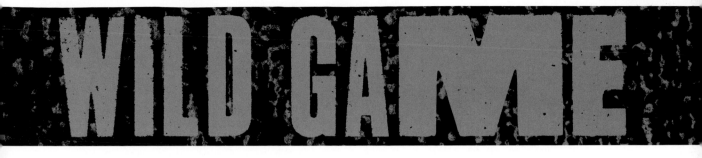

WILD GAME

4 pounds (1.8 kg) bison ribs, separated (substitute grass-fed and -finished beef ribs if you can't find bison)

Salt and freshly ground black pepper

1/2 cup (120 g) Caveman 'Cue (page 45)

BBQ BISON RIBS

WHILE THE HERDS OF BUFFALO ROAMING THE AMERICAN WEST ARE ONLY A SHADOW OF THEIR FORMER SELVES, THE ANIMAL HAS MADE A COMEBACK IN RECENT YEARS. OWING TO THE FACT THAT BISON DON'T LIKE BEING CONFINED, THEY ARE ALMOST ALWAYS PASTURE RAISED, ENSURING A MORE HUMANE EXISTENCE AND NUTRITIONALLY SUPERIOR MEAT.

Season the ribs generously with salt and pepper and wrap tightly in foil. Preheat the grill to 225°F (107°C) and wrap the ribs tightly in aluminum foil. Place the ribs over indirect heat and cook with the grill lid closed for 2 to 3 hours, turning the package of ribs every 30 minutes. The ribs are done with this phase when they are tender, but not falling off the bone, and the internal temperature reads 160°F (71°C).

Remove the foil packages from the heat and allow the ribs to rest for at least 15 minutes. Meanwhile, increase the heat on your grill, either by turning up the gas or adding more coals to the fire.

Remove the ribs from the foil and brush with the sauce. Cook the ribs over direct heat until they begin to crisp, about 3 to 4 minutes per side. Serve immediately.

YIELD: 3 OR 4 SERVINGS

"For us hunting wasn't a sport. It was a way to be intimate with nature, that intimacy providing us with wild unprocessed food free from pesticides and hormones and with the bonus of having been produced without the addition of great quantities of fossil fuel. We lived close to the animals we ate. We knew their habits and that knowledge deepened our thanks to them and the land that made them." **—TED KERASOTE,** *Merle's Door: Lessons from a Freethinking Dog*

BISON STEAKS

FOR MARINADE:

1 1/2 cups (355 ml) extra virgin olive oil

3 cloves garlic, minced

3/4 cup (180 ml) dry red wine

1 teaspoon ground black pepper

FOR STEAKS:

Six 6- to 8-ounce (168 to 225 g)
New York strip buffalo steaks

BISON MEAT IS LEANER THAN A SIMILAR CUT OF
BEEF STEAK. IT'S BEST SERVED RARE TO MEDIUM-
RARE; OTHERWISE, YOUR JAW MUSCLES WILL BE
GETTING A WORKOUT.

TO MAKE THE MARINADE: Place the olive oil and
garlic in a small bowl. While whisking, slowly add
the red wine to form an emulsion. Add the black
pepper and mix well.

TO MAKE THE STEAKS: Place the steaks in a
nonreactive pan and pour the marinade over the
meat, ensuring that each piece is evenly coated.
Cover the pan and allow the steaks to marinate in the
refrigerator for 6 to 12 hours, turning several times.

When ready to cook, remove the steaks from the
marinade and discard the marinade.

Preheat the grill to high heat. Place the steaks over
direct heat and cook for 2 to 3 minutes per side for
medium-rare. When done, the internal temperature
should be about 130°F (54°C) for medium-rare, 135°F
(57°C) for medium, 145°F (63°C) for medium-well,
and 150°F (66°C) for well. Remove the steaks from
the grill and let them rest for 5 minutes before serving.

YIELD: 6 SERVINGS

GRILLED RABBIT WITH PANCETTA, FENNEL, AND SPRING ONION

2 cloves garlic, peeled

1 small bunch fresh thyme, leaves picked from stems

1/4 teaspoon celery seed

1 tablespoon (15 ml) extra virgin olive oil

1/2 teaspoon salt

1/4 teaspoon freshly ground black pepper

2 rabbits (1/2 pound, or 227 g, each), quartered

1 bulb fresh fennel, cored and cut into 6 wedges

2 spring onions, cut in half

3-ounce (85 g) piece uncured pancetta

Juice of 1 lemon

4 or 5 sprigs Italian parsley, roughly chopped

2 tablespoons (30 ml) balsamic vinegar

Using a mortar and pestle, make a paste of the garlic,
thyme, celery seed, olive oil, salt, and pepper. Rinse
and pat dry all of the rabbit pieces. Rub the herb
paste over the rabbit pieces and place in a bowl.
Cover and refrigerate 2 to 24 hours.

Preheat your grill to medium heat with areas
providing both direct and indirect heat. Rub the
rabbit pieces with a little extra olive oil and place over
indirect heat. Cook for 8 minutes on each side.

In a medium-size bowl, toss the fennel, spring
onions, and pancetta in a drizzle of olive oil. Place on
the grill over direct heat, cooking until slightly
charred, roughly 8 minutes. Transfer the vegetables
and pancetta to a cutting board. Roughly chop the
vegetables and pancetta and transfer them to a
mixing bowl. Sprinkle with black pepper, add the
lemon juice and parsley, and stir to combine.

Spoon the vegetable/pancetta mixture over the
top, drizzle with the balsamic vinegar, and serve.

YIELD: 2 TO 4 SERVINGS

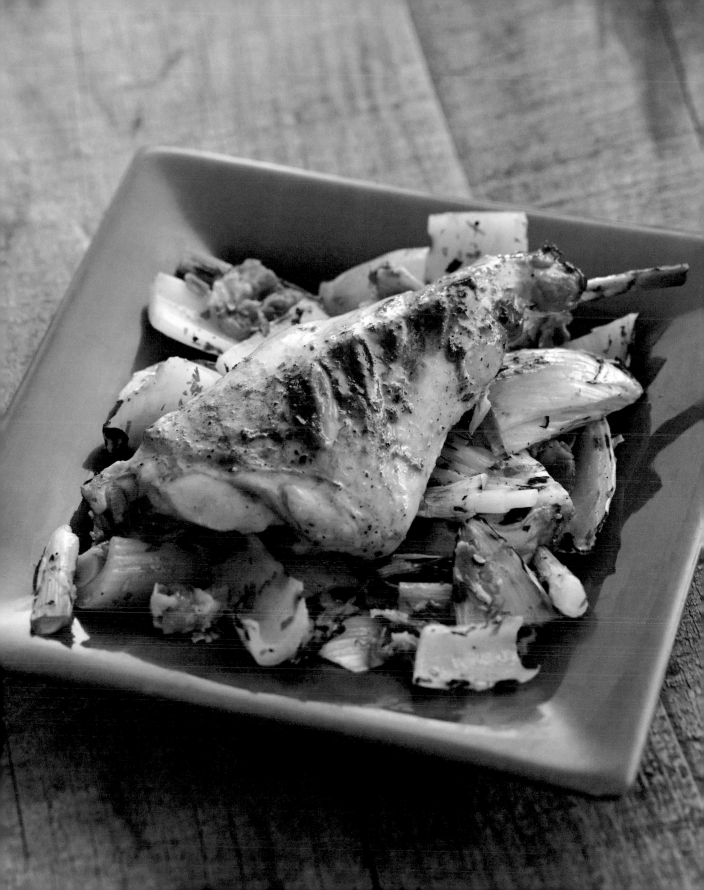

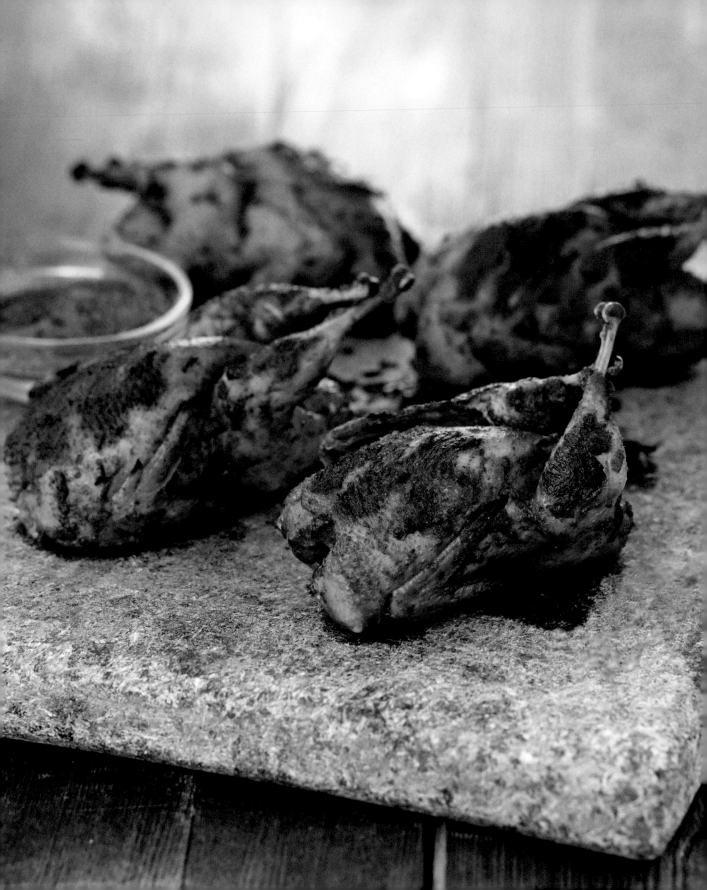

CITRUS GRILLED QUAIL

8 quail (about 5 ounces [140 g] each), cleaned

1 tablespoon (7 g) Wild Rub (page 49)

$^1/_2$ cup (120 ml) plus 1 tablespoon (15 ml) extra virgin olive oil, divided

$^1/_2$ cup (120 ml) orange juice

6 tablespoons (66 g) Dijon mustard

Sea salt

PROPERLY MARINATED AND GRILLED, QUAIL WILL HAVE AN INCREDIBLE DEEP, YET DELICATE FLAVOR. MAKE SURE YOU DO NOT OVERCOOK THESE BIRDS, OR THEY WILL BECOME DRY.

Coat the quail inside and out with the rub. Place the birds in zip-top bags and refrigerate for 1 hour.

In a small bowl, mix together $^1/_2$ cup (120 ml) of the olive oil, orange juice, and mustard. Pour half of the mixture into the bags with the quail and reserve the other half for basting later. Allow the quail to marinate in the refrigerator for 2 more hours. Remove the quail from the marinade and pat dry with paper towels.

Preheat the grill to medium heat. Rub the quail with the remaining 1 tablespoon (15 ml) olive oil and season with sea salt. Grill the birds, breast side down, over indirect heat for 8 minutes, then brush with the reserved marinade and turn over. Continue to baste the birds as they cook for an additional 7 to 10 minutes. Allow the quail to rest for 5 minutes before serving a whole bird to each guest.

YIELD: 8 SERVINGS

2 wild boar tenderloins, 8 ounces (224 g) each

1 clove garlic, cut in half

1/2 cup (86 g) Pig Rub (page 48)

1 pound (455 g) bacon

1 tablespoon (15 ml) olive oil

1/4 cup (40 g) finely diced onion

1/4 cup (38 g) diced bell pepper

1/2 cup (35 g) sliced mushrooms

1 tablespoon (11 g) Dijon mustard

1/2 cup (120 ml) beef or veal stock

SUSPECTED TO BE THE DESCENDANTS OF EUROPEAN BLACK BOARS AND ESCAPED DOMESTIC PIGS, WILD BOARS ARE CONSIDERED A NUISANCE ANIMAL AND ARE CLASSIFIED AS AN INVASIVE SPECIES ALL ACROSS THE UNITED STATES. AS A RESULT, THERE ARE FEW LIMITS ON HUNTING THEM. THEY CAN BE QUITE DANGEROUS, HOWEVER, SO IF YOU WOULD PREFER NOT TO HUNT, THERE ARE COMPANIES LIKE BROKEN ARROW RANCH (BROKENARROWRANCH.COM) THAT WILL SHIP WILD BOAR MEAT TO YOU.

Remove the silver skin from the tenderloins and rub the meat with the cut end of the garlic clove. Sprinkle the tenderloin lightly with the rub and wrap with bacon strips, using toothpicks to secure the bacon in place.

Preheat the grill to medium heat with one side providing indirect heat. Place the tenderloin over indirect heat and close the lid. Allow the meat to cook for 20 to 30 minutes, or until the internal temperature reaches 160°F (71°C). The tenderloin is done when all the bacon on the outside is thoroughly browned. Remove the tenderloin from the grill and let it rest for 5 minutes.

Heat the olive oil in a large frying pan over medium heat. Add the onion and bell pepper to the pan and cook until softened and the onions become translucent (about 5 minutes), then add the mushrooms, Dijon mustard, and beef or veal stock. Simmer for 10 minutes.

To serve, cut the tenderloin into slices while still wrapped in bacon. Arrange 2 or 3 slices per plate and top with a portion of the sautéed vegetables.

YIELD: 2 TO 4 SERVINGS

GRILLED GATOR TAIL

1 tablespoon (3.6 g) red pepper flakes

1 tablespoon (1.7 g) fresh rosemary

4 alligator tail steaks, about
$^3/_4$ inch (2 cm) thick

$^1/_2$ teaspoon freshly ground black pepper

$^1/_4$ teaspoon cayenne pepper

1 can (14 ounces, or 425 ml) full-fat coconut milk

1 cup (100 g) Wild Rub (page 49)

Olive oil, for drizzling

WHILE IT DOESN'T EXACTLY "TASTE LIKE CHICKEN," GATOR MEAT DOES HAVE A TENDENCY TO BE TOUGH IF HANDLED IMPROPERLY. FLAVOR IT UP WITH A GREAT MARINADE AND COOK IT HOT AND FAST TO KEEP IT TENDER AND TASTY.

Put the red pepper flakes and rosemary in a large bowl. Season the alligator meat with the black and cayenne peppers and put the meat into the bowl with the spices. Pour the coconut milk over the top of the meat, cover the bowl, and let it marinate in the refrigerator for 3 to 4 hours.

Preheat the grill to high heat. Remove the meat from the marinade and discard the marinade. Pat the meat dry and season generously with the rub. Drizzle with olive oil to reduce sticking, and grill the steaks over direct heat for 10 minutes per side. The gator tail is done when the meat is white in the center and the juices run clear. Don't overcook or the meat will become tough.

YIELD: 4 SERVINGS

PEPPERCORN-CRUSTED VENISON BACKSTRAP

3 tablespoons (15 g) black peppercorns

1 tablespoon (5 g) coriander seed

3 tablespoons (15 g) juniper berries

4 tablespoons (10 g) fresh thyme leaves

1 teaspoon sea salt

1 tablespoon (15 ml) extra virgin olive oil

2 venison loins or backstraps (1$^1/_2$ pounds, or 680 g, each), trimmed

VENISON BACKSTRAP IS SOMETIMES REFERRED TO AS THE "FILET MIGNON" OF DEER. THE MEAT IS PRIZED FOR ITS LEAN, RICH TEXTURE AND FOR THE FACT THAT VENISON IS NATURALLY ANTIBIOTIC AND HORMONE FREE.

Using a spice grinder or mortar and pestle, coarsely grind the peppercorns, coriander, and juniper berries. Transfer the spices to a small mixing bowl and combine with the thyme, sea salt, and olive oil. Rub the venison backstraps thoroughly with the mixture, wrap them in plastic wrap, and refrigerate for 1 to 2 hours.

Preheat the grill to high heat. Place the backstraps over direct heat, grill for 4 to 5 minutes, turn 90 degrees, and cook for 5 minutes longer, then flip and repeat the process on the other side. The venison is done when the spices and herbs on the outside are charred but the center of the meat is still rare. Allow the meat to rest for 10 to 12 minutes before serving.

When ready to serve, slice the meat against the grain.

YIELD: 8 TO 10 SERVINGS

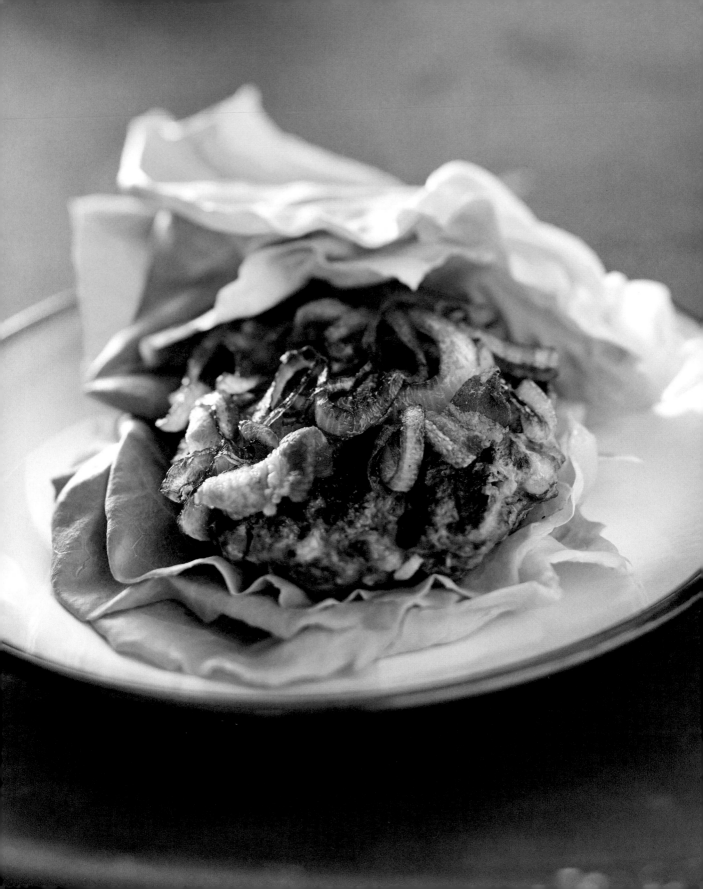

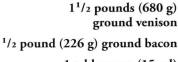

DOUBLE BACON BAMBI BURGERS

1¹/₂ pounds (680 g)
ground venison

¹/₂ pound (226 g) ground bacon

1 tablespoon (15 ml)
Worcestershire sauce

2 teaspoons (4 g) freshly
ground black pepper

2 teaspoons (12 g) sea salt

2 tablespoons (20 g)
minced white onion

2 cloves garlic, minced

1 egg yolk

12 strips bacon

1 white onion, thinly sliced

1 large head iceberg lettuce

DEPENDING ON THE AGE, DIET, AND SEX OF THE DEER, THE "GAMINESS" OF VENISON MEAT CAN VARY WILDLY. AN OLD HUNTER'S TRICK IS TO ADD A SPLASH OF WORCESTERSHIRE SAUCE TO GROUND VENISON TO BOTH FLAVOR THE MEAT AND HIDE ANY GAMINESS THAT MIGHT BE PRESENT.

In a large bowl, combine the ground venison, ground bacon, Worcestershire, black pepper, salt, minced onion, garlic, and egg yolk, mixing thoroughly. Form the meat mixture into 4 to 6 patties.

In a sauté pan, cook the bacon over medium-high heat until browned. Transfer to a paper towel–lined plate or cooling rack and leave the rendered bacon fat in the pan. Add the sliced onion to the pan and cook until caramelized, approximately 20 minutes. Reduce the heat to low to keep the onions warm.

Preheat the grill to high heat. Cook the burgers over direct heat for 5 to 6 minutes, flip, then cook for 3 to 5 minutes longer, or until desired doneness. Top with the bacon and caramelized onions and serve in an iceberg lettuce wrap.

YIELD: 4 TO 6 SERVINGS

GRILLED PHEASANT BREAST

2 cups (470 ml) balsamic vinegar

2 cups (470 ml) Calvados or regular brandy

6 dried juniper berries

2 tablespoons (10 g) coriander seed

3 sprigs fresh thyme, cut in half

1 sprig fresh rosemary, cut in half

1 sprig fresh oregano, cut in half

1 sprig fresh tarragon, cut in half

1 cup (235 ml) extra virgin olive oil

6 boneless pheasant breasts

PHEASANTS ARE SMALLER THAN CHICKENS AND
CAN FLY WELL, A FACT THAT MAKES THEIR
BREAST MEAT RICHER AND MORE FLAVORFUL.

In a medium saucepot over medium heat, combine
the balsamic vinegar, Calvados, juniper berries,
coriander seed, and herbs. When it starts to simmer,
turn off the heat and allow the mixture to return to
room temperature. When cool, strain through a fine
sieve into a mixing bowl. Whisk in the olive oil and
then place the pheasant breasts into the bowl. Cover
and refrigerate for 6 to 12 hours.

Preheat the grill to medium heat. Remove the
pheasant breasts from the marinade and discard the
marinade. Place the pheasant breasts, skin side
down, over direct heat and close the lid. Allow the
pheasant to cook for 6 to 8 minutes, then flip and
cook for an additional 3 minutes on the other side,
or until the pheasant reaches an internal temperature
of 140ºF (60ºC). Remove from the grill and allow to
rest for 8 minutes before slicing.

YIELD: 6 SERVINGS

VENISON BROCHETTES

FOR MARINADE:

$^3/_4$ cup (180 ml) olive oil

3 tablespoons (7.5 g) chopped fresh basil

2 tablespoons (30 ml) lemon juice
1 tablespoon (3.5 g) red pepper flakes

FOR VENISON BROCHETTES:

2 red or green bell peppers

1 teaspoon olive oil

2-pound (907 g) venison leg or shoulder roast, cut
into 1 $^1/_2$-inch (3.8 cm) cubes

4 baby artichokes, cut in half

Black pepper to taste

Preheat the grill to high heat.

TO MAKE THE MARINADE: Combine the ingredients in a large bowl. Reserve one-fourth of the marinade.

TO MAKE THE VENISON BROCHETTES: Rub the
bell peppers with olive oil and cook over direct heat
until blackened, about 8 minutes. Place the peppers
in a bowl and cover with plastic wrap. After 2 to 3
minutes, remove the bell peppers and rub them
vigorously to remove most of the charred skin. Cut
the peppers into large chunks and return to the bowl.

Add the chunks of venison, artichokes, and
marinade to the bowl. Lightly toss to coat all of the
ingredients and allow to sit for 30 minutes before
threading onto skewers.

Season the skewers with black pepper and grill
over direct high heat for 2 to 3 minutes, basting with
the reserved marinade. Turn the skewers and cook for
an additional 2 to 3 minutes while continuing to
baste with the marinade. When done, the venison
should be rare, with an internal temperature of about
125°F (52°C).

YIELD: 6 SERVINGS

GRILLED OSTRICH FLANK WITH BLACKBERRY–BLOOD ORANGE SAUCE

FOR BLACKBERRY–BLOOD ORANGE SAUCE:

2 cups (470 ml) freshly squeezed blood orange juice (you can use premade juice if fresh oranges are not available)

1 tablespoon (12 g) coconut sugar

2 tablespoons (30 ml) apple cider vinegar

2 cups (290 g) fresh blackberries (frozen, defrosted blackberries can be substituted)

2 tablespoons (3.4 g) chopped fresh rosemary

FOR OSTRICH:

4 ostrich steaks (5 to 6 ounces [140 to 170 g] each)

Sea salt

Black pepper

Garlic powder

Olive oil

OSTRICH MEAT IS A GREAT "STARTER" MEAT FOR THOSE WHO ARE INTIMIDATED BY EATING OUTSIDE OF THE CHICKEN, PIG, BEEF TRIUMVIRATE. OSTRICH IS HIGH IN PROTEIN AND IRON, BUT LOW IN CALORIES AND FAT. IT HAS A SUPER RICH TEXTURE AND IS NOT GAMEY IN THE LEAST.

TO MAKE THE SAUCE: In a small pot, heat the blood orange juice, coconut sugar, and apple cider vinegar over medium heat until the mixture starts to bubble. Whisk the sauce well and add the blackberries and rosemary. Turn off the heat, stir, and cover the pot with a lid. Set the sauce aside.

TO MAKE THE OSTRICH: Preheat your grill to high heat. Season the ostrich steaks with a dusting of salt, black pepper, and garlic powder. Drizzle the meat with olive oil and place over direct high heat. Sear the steaks for 2 minutes, turn the meat 90 degrees, cook for another 2 minutes, flip the steaks, and repeat the process on the other side. Remove the steaks from the grill while they are still rare and transfer to a cutting board. Let the meat rest for 5 to 8 minutes before slicing it thinly against the grain.

To serve, transfer the slices to a platter and spoon the sauce lightly over them.

YIELD: 4 SERVINGS

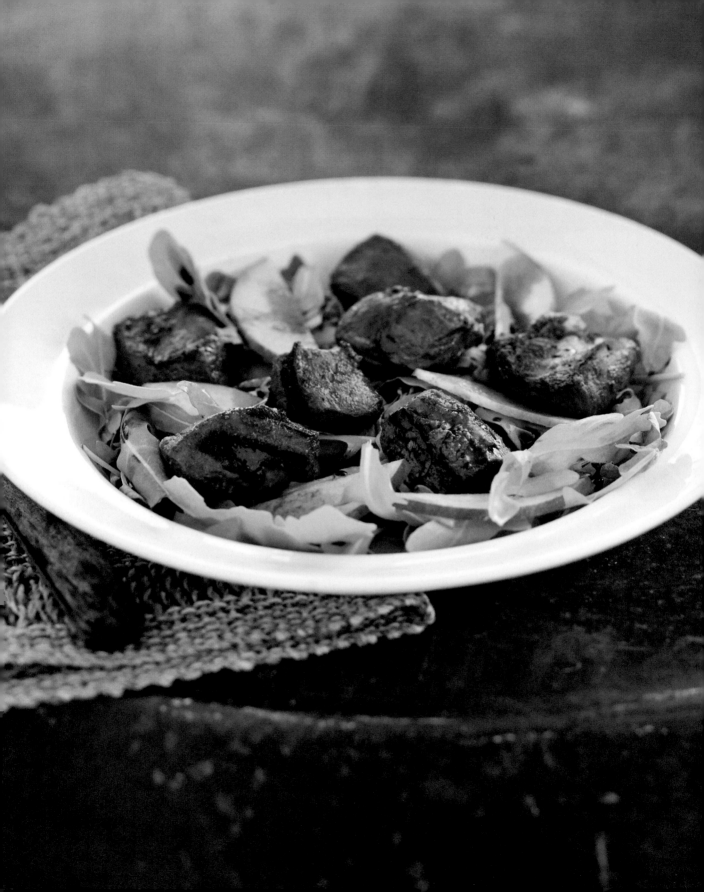

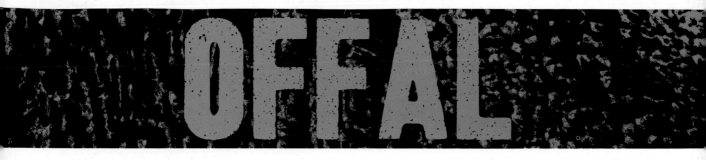

2 teaspoons (5 g) sweet paprika

1 teaspoon ground cumin

$^1/_2$ teaspoon cayenne pepper

$^1/_2$ teaspoon dark chili powder

$1^1/_2$ teaspoons (9 g) sea salt

Juice of $^1/_2$ orange

Zest of 1 orange

1 tablespoon (14 g) coconut oil, melted

$1^1/_2$ pounds (680 g) lamb hearts

20 leaves arugula

$^1/_2$ peach, thinly sliced

Balsamic vinegar (look for Aceto Balsamico Tradizionale; this is the real stuff aged for 10 years in oak barrels)

Extra virgin olive oil

MOROCCAN LAMB HEART KEBABS

HEART, UNLIKE OTHER FORMS OF OFFAL, IS REALLY JUST ANOTHER MUSCLE. IT HAS A UNIQUE TEXTURE BECAUSE THE FIBERS ARE ARRANGED DIFFERENTLY, BUT THE FLAVOR IS QUITE FAMILIAR. ADDITIONALLY, HEART IS A GREAT SOURCE FOR MANY VITAMINS AND MINERALS, SUCH AS NIACIN, PHOSPHORUS, ZINC, IRON, SELENIUM, RIBOFLAVIN, AND B_{12}.

Soak six 6-inch (15 cm) wooden skewers in water for at least 1 hour (or use metal skewers).

Combine the paprika, cumin, cayenne, chili powder, salt, orange juice, orange zest, and coconut oil in a mixing bowl and set aside. Clean the lamb's heart by removing the top part that contains the fat and valves. Cut open the first chamber and lay it flat, cleaning the thick tissue and strings away from the heart. Do the same for the second chamber, cutting away thick or hard tissue. Cut the heart into 1-inch (2.5 cm) cubes. Place the cubes in the bowl with the spice mixture and rub thoroughly. Cover in plastic and allow to marinate for 1 to 3 hours in the refrigerator.

When ready to cook, preheat your grill to high heat and remove the lamb heart from the refrigerator. Thread the marinated heart cubes onto the skewers and grill for 1 minute per side. Repeat until all sides are cooked. Remove from the grill and serve hot over the arugula. Garnish with the peach slices and drizzle with the aged balsamic vinegar and olive oil.

YIELD: 6 SERVINGS

"Understand, when you eat meat, that something did die. You have an obligation to value it—not just the sirloin but also all those wonderful tough little bits." **—ANTHONY BOURDAIN**

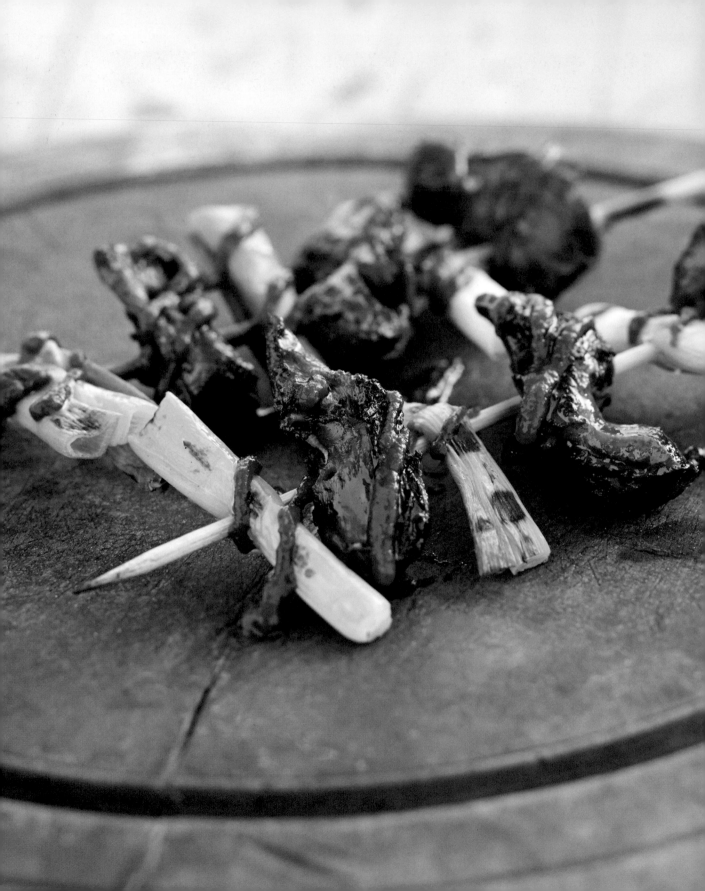

BARBECUED CHICKEN GIZZARD YAKITORI

1 pound (454 g) chicken gizzards, cleaned and butterflied

2 cups (470 ml) Soy-Free Soy Sauce–Style Meat Marinade (page 53)

8 scallions, cut into 2-inch (5 cm) pieces, roots and top green sections removed (save these for garnish)

Fresh lime slices

Sriracha chili sauce

YAKITORI VENDORS SELLING SKEWERED MEATS COOKED OVER AN OPEN FLAME ARE A COMMON SIGHT IN JAPAN. ALL PARTS OF THE ANIMAL ARE USED, INCLUDING THE GIZZARD, A MUSCULAR ORGAN THAT BIRDS USE TO HELP DIGEST THEIR FOOD. SLOW COOKING THE GIZZARDS BEFORE GRILLING TENDERIZES AND FLAVORS THE MEAT, KEEPING IT FROM BECOMING OVERLY TOUGH.

Soak 8 wooden skewers in water for at least 1 hour (or use metal skewers).

In a saucepan, combine the chicken gizzards and marinade. Bring to a boil over high heat, lower the heat to a simmer, cover, and cook for 45 minutes. Keep an eye on the liquid level, adding just enough water (about $1/2$ cup [120 ml] at a time) to prevent the gizzards from burning. Transfer the gizzards to a plate and let cool.

Preheat your grill to high heat. Thread 3 gizzards onto each skewer, alternating with the scallion pieces. Cook the skewers over direct heat for approximately 4 minutes, flip, and cook for 3 to 4 minutes longer. Garnish with the tops of the scallion, fresh lime slices, and a drizzle of sriracha.

YIELD: 8 SERVINGS

AWESOME SMOKED OFFAL MEATLOAF

1 egg, beaten

2 shallots, minced

1 Anaheim chile, seeded and diced

1¹/₄ cups (285 g) Kicked-Up Ketchup (page 46), divided

2 teaspoons (4 g) black pepper

2 teaspoons (5 g) granulated garlic

1 teaspoon fennel seed

4 sprigs thyme, leaves picked and chopped

¹/₂ cup (60 g) almond flour

¹/₂ pound (227 g) ground beef heart

¹/₂ pound (227 g) pureed beef liver

¹/₂ pound (227 g) ground beef

¹/₂ pound (227 g) ground pork bacon

5 pounds (2.3 kg) mesquite wood chunks

ORGAN MEATS SUCH AS LIVER ARE TRUE "SUPERFOODS," RICH IN BIOAVAILABLE VITAMINS AND MINERALS SUCH AS IRON. UNLESS YOU GREW UP EATING THEM, HOWEVER, THEIR UNFAMILIAR FLAVOR AND TEXTURE CAN BE OFF-PUTTING. BLENDING OFFAL SUCH AS BEEF HEART AND LIVER WITH MORE POPULAR MEATS SUCH AS GROUND BEEF AND BACON HELPS DISGUISE THEIR FLAVOR WHILE MAINTAINING THEIR NUTRITIONAL BENEFITS. THIS PARTICULAR RECIPE, MIXED WITH HERBS, GLAZED WITH KICKED-UP KETCHUP, AND SMOKED ON THE GRILL OR IN THE SMOKER, PRODUCES A RICH FLAVOR THAT IS SIMPLY AWESOME.

In a large mixing bowl, combine the egg, shallots, Anaheim chile, ¹/₄ cup (60 g) of the ketchup, black pepper, granulated garlic, fennel seed, thyme, and almond flour. Mix with a rubber spatula into a thick paste. Add the ground heart, liver, beef, and bacon and mix thoroughly. Pour the meatloaf mixture into the center of a disposable aluminum cooking pan, forming a loose mound.

Preheat the grill with the coals set off to one side. When the internal temperature reaches 250ºF (120ºC), add 3 mesquite chunks on top of the coals. If you are using a gas grill, put the wood in a smoker box over direct heat.

Put the pan with the meatloaf over indirect heat and close the lid. Adjust the top and bottom vents and add more coals/wood as needed to maintain a temperature of 225ºF (107ºC) inside the grill. Smoke the meatloaf for 3 to 4 hours, or until the center reaches 160°F (71ºC). About 30 minutes before the meatloaf is finished, baste it with the remaining 1 cup (240 g) Kicked-Up Ketchup to form the glaze.

YIELD: 8 SERVINGS

GRILLED SWEETBREADS WITH AJO BLANCO

11$^{1}/_{2}$ ounces (322 g) soaked
and blanched sweetbreads

Olive oil

Black pepper

1 cup (260 g) Ajo Blanco (page 47)

SWEETBREADS ARE ACTUALLY THE THYMUS GLAND OF A YOUNG COW. SWEETBREADS HAVE A UNIQUELY SOFT TEXTURE FOR AN ORGAN MEAT AND A MUCH MILDER FLAVOR THAN OTHER OFFAL.

Preheat the grill to medium-high heat.

When selecting your sweetbreads, make sure they smell clean, are a pale white in color, and don't have a lot of blood. Before starting any preparation with them, soak them in heavily salted water for 4 to 6 hours, draining and refreshing the water a couple of times during the process. This will extract the excess blood and impurities that may be present. They also should be blanched in salted boiling water for 2 minutes and then shocked in ice water. This will firm the texture and make it easier to remove the outer membrane.

Using a paring knife, trim the outer tough membrane from the sweetbreads. Be sure to leave the thin membrane intact so that it stays together. Place the sweetbreads on a cutting board and slice them lengthwise about halfway through. Open them like a book, rub with olive oil, and season with black pepper. Place on the grill open side down. Grill for 6 to 8 minutes, flip over, and grill for 6 to 8 more minutes. They should have an internal temperature of 145°F (63°C). Remove from the grill and allow to cool for 5 minutes. Slice into medallions and top with the sauce.

YIELD: 2 TO 4 SERVINGS

GRILLED LAMB LIVER MEATBALLS

8-ounce (224 g) lamb or calf liver,
cut into small pieces

1 pound (454 g) ground beef

2 teaspoons (5 g) cumin

1 teaspoon smoked paprika

1 teaspoon sea salt

1 teaspoon black pepper

$^{1}/_{2}$ teaspoon ground thyme

2 tablespoons (30 ml) lemon juice

2 tablespoons (30 ml) olive oil

THIS IS A SNEAKY WAY TO GET THE HEALTH BENEFITS OF LIVER WITHOUT TURNING OFF FRIENDS OR FAMILY WHO MIGHT NOT BE GAME. THE GROUND BEEF PROVIDES A FAMILIAR TEXTURE WHILE LAMB LIVER'S NATURALLY MILD FLAVOR IS HARDLY NOTICEABLE.

Mix the liver, ground meat, spices, lemon juice, and oil together in a bowl. Run the mixture through your meat grinder and form into meatballs the size of golf balls. If you don't have a meat grinder, you can puree the liver in a blender or food processor before mixing it by hand with the other ingredients.

Preheat your grill to high heat. Grill the meatballs over direct high heat for approximately 4 minutes. Flip and cook for an additional 4 minutes. Serve medium-rare (internal temperature of 145°F [63°C]).

YIELD: 4 OR 5 SERVINGS

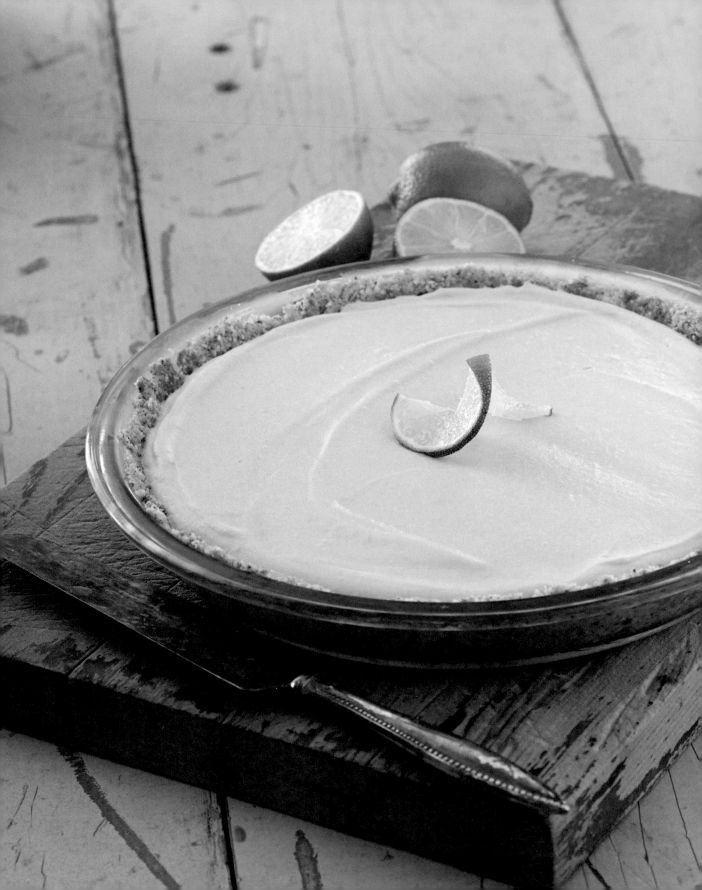

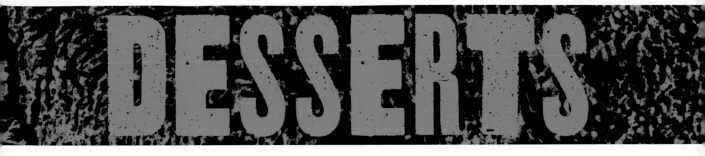

DESSERTS

FOR CRUST:

2 tablespoons (30 g) coconut butter

6 Medjool dates

1 cup (110 g) toasted almond slices

¹/₂ cup (40 g) unsweetened coconut flakes

¹/₂ teaspoon vanilla extract

Pinch of salt

FOR FILLING:

2 ripe avocados

¹/₂ cup (120 ml) freshly squeezed lime juice

¹/₃ cup (80 ml) maple syrup

1 to 2 tablespoons (8 to 16 g) coconut flour

2 cans (14 ounces, or 425 ml, each) full-fat coconut milk, chilled

PALEO KEY LIME PIE

THERE WEREN'T PIES IN THE PALEOLITHIC AGE, BUT IT'S HARD TO IMAGINE ANY REASONABLE CAVEMAN (OR CAVEWOMAN) TURNING DOWN THIS RENDITION OF THE CLASSIC DESSERT. THE RECIPE COMES COURTESY OF ROSE FROM THECLEANDISH.COM.

TO MAKE THE CRUST: Melt the coconut butter in a skillet over low heat, being careful not to let it burn. In a food processor, pulse the dates for 1 to 2 minutes. Add the almond slices and coconut flakes and process again for 1 to 2 minutes. Add the melted coconut butter, vanilla, and salt and process until sticky and crumbly. Press the crust into a pie dish and refrigerate.

TO MAKE THE FILLING: Peel the avocados and place in a food processor together with the lime juice, maple syrup, and coconut flour. Process until smooth and thick.

Carefully remove the coconut milk from the refrigerator and scoop out the cream at the top. Beat the cream in a bowl until it reaches the consistency of whipped cream. Fold the avocado mixture into the coconut cream and continue to beat until well incorporated. Pour the filling into the prepared pie crust and place in the freezer for 2 to 3 hours, or until the center is firm. Transfer to the refrigerator and chill for another 2 hours before serving.

YIELD: 6 TO 8 SERVINGS

NOT ALL COCONUT MILK IS MADE THE SAME

Look for Native Forest or Arroy-D brands of full-fat coconut milk. They are BPA-free and, when refrigerated, quickly separate into rich coconut cream that is perfect for this recipe.

"Life is uncertain. Eat dessert first."
—ERNESTINE ULMER

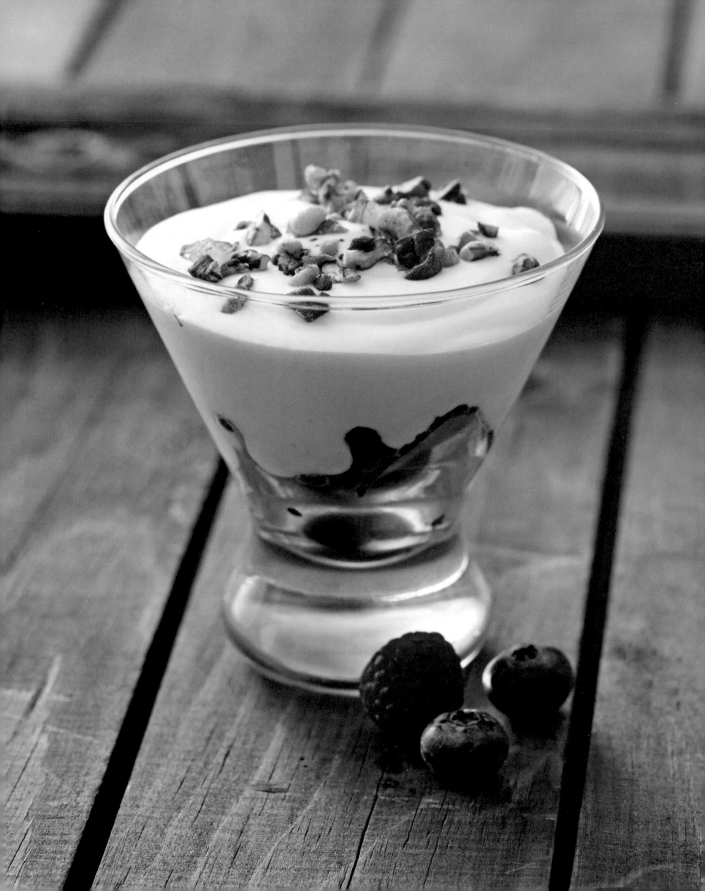

MIXED BERRY PARFAIT

2 cups (250 g) mixed berries (blueberries, blackberries, sliced strawberries, raspberries, etc.)

1 can (14 ounces, or 425 ml) full-fat coconut milk, chilled

Toasted nuts (almonds, pecans, etc.), for topping

Cinnamon, for sprinkling

THERE IS NOTHING BETTER THAN A PERFECTLY RIPE BLUEBERRY, RASPBERRY, OR BLACKBERRY. WILD-HARVESTED VARIETIES ARE RICHER IN FLAVOR AND HAVE HIGHER LEVELS OF BIOFLAVONOIDS AND OTHER HEALTHFUL COMPOUNDS. IF ALL THE BERRIES LISTED IN THIS RECIPE AREN'T IN SEASON WHERE YOU LIVE, STICK WITH WHATEVER YOU CAN FIND LOCALLY.

Divide the mixed berries among 4 small glass or dessert dishes. Open the can of coconut milk and scoop out the cream that has accumulated at the top. In a bowl with a hand mixer or a whisk, beat the coconut cream until fluffy. Top each parfait with coconut cream and sprinkle with toasted nuts and a pinch of cinnamon.

YIELD: 4 SERVINGS

GETTIN' TOASTED

To toast nuts, simply smash them up by putting them in a heavy-duty zip-top bag and crushing with a heavy rolling pin or mallet. Put the crushed nuts on a cookie sheet and toast in a 300°F (150°C, or gas mark 2) oven for approximately 5 minutes. Keep a close eye on them to ensure they don't burn.

CHUNKY CHOCOLATE BANANA POPS

8 wooden ice pop sticks

4 medium-size semi-ripe bananas, peeled and cut in half

4 ounces (112 g) dairy-free, soy-free, semisweet or dark chocolate chips

¹/₃ cup (80 ml) coconut oil

TOPPING OPTIONS:

Bacon, cooked crispy and crumbled

Crushed toasted nuts (almonds, pecans, pistachios, cashews, etc.)

Shredded coconut

Chocolate chips

Raisins

BANANA POPS ARE EASY TO MAKE AND FUN TO EAT. THIS IS A GREAT PROJECT TO GET THE KIDS INVOLVED WITH, AND YOU WON'T FEEL GUILTY IF YOU END UP EATING THEM AS WELL.

Insert the Popsicle sticks into the cut ends of the banana pieces (if you don't have Popsicle sticks, you can simply cut each banana into bite-size pieces and make "bites" instead of "pops"). Place the bananas on a cookie sheet lined with parchment paper and place in the freezer to harden, about 30 minutes.

Melt the chocolate chips in a double boiler over medium heat (if you don't have a double boiler, a small pot set inside a larger pot with some water in it will do, just be sure to avoid getting any water into the melting chocolate). When the chocolate has melted, mix with the coconut oil.

One by one, take a frozen banana pop and dip it into the chocolate mixture, ensuring that it is evenly coated. Quickly roll the banana pop in the topping of choice and put it back onto the parchment-lined cookie sheet. When all of the banana pops are finished, put them back in the freezer for another 15 to 30 minutes before serving.

The finished pops can be stored for a week in the freezer, but if they are hard-frozen, put them in the refrigerator for 30 minutes to soften before serving.

YIELD: 8 SERVINGS

"There's nothing better than a good friend, except a good friend with chocolate." —**LINDA GRAYSON**

WATERMELON MOJITO FREEZER SORBET

THIS "ADULTS ONLY" DESSERT IS SURE TO PLEASE AFTER A HOT DAY OF TENDING THE GRILL.

4 cups (600 g) chopped seedless watermelon

1 cup (96 g) fresh mint leaves

¼ cup (60 ml) light rum

2 cups (470 ml) coconut water

Juice of 2 limes

Place the watermelon, mint, rum, coconut water, and lime juice in a blender and blend until completely puréed. Pour the mixture into a 10 x 12-inch (25 x 30.5 cm) baking dish. Put into the freezer and allow to chill for 1½ hours. Remove the pan and scrape the ice with a fork, being sure to mix the softer center with the more frozen outer edges. Return the pan to the freezer for another 1½ hours. Before serving, scrape again using the fork.

YIELD: 6 TO 8 SERVINGS

GRILLED PEACHES WITH COCONUT ICE CREAM

PEACHES ON THE GRILL CARAMELIZE AND INTENSIFY IN FLAVOR. HOT GRILLED PEACHES PAIRED WITH A COLD COCONUT MILK ICE CREAM LITERALLY MELT IN YOUR MOUTH.

FOR VANILLA COCONUT ICE CREAM:

2 cans (14 ounces, or 425 ml, each) full-fat coconut milk, chilled

1 teaspoon vanilla extract

Pinch of sea salt

Pinch of cinnamon, plus more for garnish

1 tablespoon (15 ml) coconut nectar

FOR PEACHES:

4 ripe peaches, cut in half and pitted

1 tablespoon (14 g) coconut oil, melted

TO MAKE THE COCONUT MILK ICE CREAM: Remove the coconut cream layer from both cans of coconut milk and put it into a bowl. Add all of the remaining ingredients to the bowl and whisk thoroughly to incorporate air into the mixture. Pour the mixture into an ice cream maker and churn according to the manufacturer's directions until it becomes semisolid. Put the ice cream into a sealable container and place in the freezer until firm (at least 30 minutes).

TO MAKE THE PEACHES: Preheat the grill to medium-high heat. Coat the cut sides of the peaches with coconut oil and grill, cut side down, for 3 to 5 minutes. Move the peaches to the top rack of the grill, placing them skin side down. Close the lid and allow the peaches to cook for 5 to 10 minutes. When done, the peaches will be soft but not falling apart. Top each peach with a scoop of ice cream, sprinkle with cinnamon, and serve.

YIELD: 8 SERVINGS

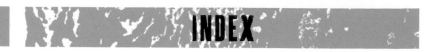

FatWorks: Purveyors of high-quality lard, tallow, and duck fat (fatworks.wazala.com)

Kasandrinos Extra Virgin Olive Oil: 100% pure Greek olive oil (kasandrinos.com)

Kombucha Mama: Oregon's finest kombucha tea (kombuchamama.com)

Wild Mountain Paleo: A one-stop shop for Paleo food products, books, and more (wildmountainpaleo.com)

U.S. Wellness Meats: Suppliers of a wide variety of beef, pork, chicken, and other meat products (grasslandbeef.com)

Lava Lake Lamb: Specialists in sustainably produced and range-fed lamb (lavalakelamb.com)

Tendergrass Farms: Grass-fed steaks and dry-aged ground beef, chicken, and pork chops from small family farms (grassfedbeef.org)

Broken Arrow Ranch: Ethically harvested and truly wild venison, boar, and antelope (brokenarrowranch.com)

INDEX

173

INDEX

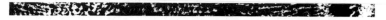

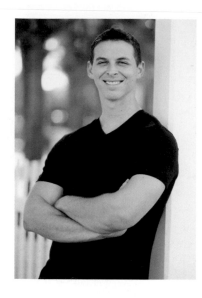

Tony Federico graduated from the University of Florida's School of Exercise and Sports Science with a bachelor's degree in applied physiology and kinesiology and has worked full-time as a personal trainer, fitness consultant, and nutrition coach since 2006. While following the conventional recommendations of "low-fat," "high-fiber," and "whole grain" eating, he was plagued with food cravings and had to constantly work out to maintain his weight. In January 2011, he discovered Paleo and, after experiencing relief from a lifetime of food struggles, has never looked back. In addition to his work as a personal trainer, Tony is a regular contributor to *Paleo Magazine* and the host of the *Paleo Magazine* radio podcast. Tony has been a presenter and panelist at events such as the Ancestral Health Symposium and PaleoFX and blogs about Paleo food and fitness at LiveCaveman.com. He currently lives in Jacksonville, Florida, with his wife, Jamie.

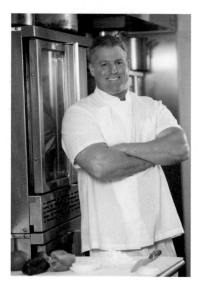

James "Jay" Phelan is a graduate of the French Culinary Institute in New York City and has served as executive chef at the AAA "Four Diamonds"–awarded Restaurant Medure (Ponte Vedra, Florida) and Matthew's Restaurant (Jacksonville, Florida). Over the years, James noticed many gym-goers struggling with their diets, either eating bland, redundant foods or regularly "cheating." He knew he could create meals that would remedy these issues and allow people to fully reap the benefits of their hard work, so in March 2011, James left the restaurant industry and started J. William Culinary, a gourmet meal delivery service. J. William Culinary provides healthy, fresh fitness meals, including many gluten-free and Paleo options. To see what's on the menu, visit Jwilliamculinary.com.